Reconstructive Surgery - Techniques and Advances

Edited by Kiran Mahapure
and Andrej Čretnik

Published in London, United Kingdom

Reconstructive Surgery - Techniques and Advances
http://dx.doi.org/10.5772/intechopen.1008020
Edited by Kiran Mahapure and Andrej Čretnik

Contributors
Alba Mayra Padilla, Ashok Marudanayagam, Celina Verónica Kishi, Dongli Fan, Francesco Benazzo, Heriberto Contreras, Ioan-Constantin Pop, Jingjun Wei, Karla Elizabeth Rincón, Loris Perticarini, Luca Andriollo, Maximilian-Vlad Muntean, Maximiliano Sánchez, Meshal Alhadhoud, Mohamed Elnemr, Pablo Meneses, Pan You, Radu-Alexandru Ilies, Ramani Saradha, Rizwan Shahid, Samarth Gupta, Sedeek M. Mosaid, Shilpi Karmakar, Shuqing Huang, Tawheed Ahmad, Venkat Ramakrishnan, Xiaohua Shi, Xin Zhou, Zeyuan Lei

First published in London, United Kingdom, 2026 by IntechOpen
IntechOpen is the global imprint of INTECHOPEN LIMITED, registered in England and Wales, registration number: 11086078, 167-169 Great Portland Street, London, W1W 5PF, United Kingdom

For EU product safety concerns: IN TECH d.o.o., Prolaz Marije Krucifikse Kozulić 3, 51000 Rijeka, Croatia, info@intechopen.com or visit our website at intechopen.com.

British Library Cataloguing-in-Publication Data
A catalogue record for this book is available from the British Library

Reconstructive Surgery - Techniques and Advances
Edited by Kiran Mahapure and Andrej Čretnik
p. cm.
Print ISBN 978-1-83635-091-0
Online ISBN 978-1-83635-090-3
eBook (PDF) ISBN 978-1-83635-092-7

If disposing of this product, please recycle the paper responsibly.

Meet the editor

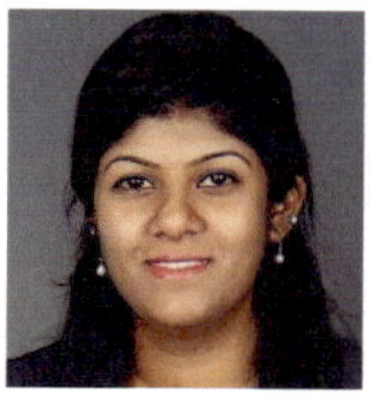

Dr. Kiran Mahapure is a board-certified plastic surgeon from India, currently pursuing higher training in breast and body contouring in the United States. Her clinical expertise spans a broad range of reconstructive and aesthetic procedures, including breast reconstruction, microsurgery, body contouring, craniofacial surgery, hand surgery, and trauma and burn reconstruction. In addition to his surgical practice, Dr. Mahapure is deeply engaged in academic medicine. She serves as a peer reviewer for over 10 international journals and is the review editor for a peer-reviewed journal. She has also co-edited a book on reconstructive surgery, advancing evidence-based surgical education and practice. Dr. Mahapure combines a solid foundation in clinical excellence with a strong commitment to academic scholarship, making her a valuable contributor to editorial and publishing initiatives in the field of plastic and reconstructive surgery. As a dedicated clinician and researcher, she brings both technical depth and a commitment to evidence-based practice to her editorial role.

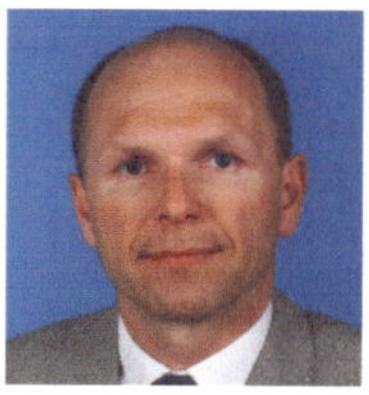

Prof. Andrej Čretnik, MD, Ph.D., Med. Councilor was born in 1963 in Celje, Slovenia. He graduated from the Medical Faculty of the University of Ljubljana, Slovenia (1989). Dr. Čretnik earned a Master of Science (MSc) in 1999 (University of Ljubljana, Slovenia) and a Doctor of Sciences (Ph.D.) (Medical Sciences) in 2002 (University of Ljubljana, Slovenia). His additional education includes the Royal Liverpool University Hospital (GB, 1994) (Foot and Ankle Surgery, Hip Surgery); Mayo Clinic, Rochester, Minnesota (USA, 1996) (Spinal Surgery); Parkland Memorial Hospital, Dallas, Texas (USA, 1996) (Pelvic Surgery); Trauma Shock Center, Baltimore, Maryland (USA, 1999) (Orthopaedic Trauma Surgery); Health Science Center, University of Texas, Houston (USA, 2002) (Orthopaedic Trauma Surgery). He is the Head of the Department of Traumatology at the Surgical Clinic of the University Clinical Center Maribor, Slovenia. Dr. Čretnik has been a Medicolegal Expert at the Ministry of Justice in Slovenia since 2004 and a Medical Councilor (2008) at the Ministry of Health, Slovenia, since 2008. He is a member of the Medical Chamber of Slovenia, Slovene Medical Association, Slovene Trauma Association (past-president), Slovene Medicolegal Experts Association, SQAA (Slovenia, National Evaluator), and the European Society for Trauma and Emergency Surgery (ESTES), AO Trauma Society & AO Faculty (Arbeitsgruppe für Osteosynthesefragen, Davos, CH), past chairman of Quality Assurance Committee (Medical Faculty, University of Maribor, Slovenia), and current chairman of Medicolegal Experts Committee (Medical Faculty, University of Maribor, Slovenia).

Contents

Preface

This Edited Volume is a collection of reviewed and relevant research chapters on developments in the field of Reconstructive Surgery. The book includes scholarly contributions from various authors and is edited by experts in the field. Each contribution comes as a separate chapter complete in itself but directly related to the book's topics and objectives.

The book includes the following chapters:

1. New Strategies for Prevention and Treatment of Sternal Wound Infection: Clinical Big Data-Driven Prediction and Precision Diagnosis-Treatment Integrated System in Plastic Surgery

2. Evolution and Innovation in Reconstructive Breast Surgery: A Comprehensive Review

3. A Structured Approach to DIEP Flap Reconstruction: Imaging, Execution, and Handling Surgical Challenges

4. Tendon Surgery for Thigh Injury in Professional Football Players

5. Achilles Tendon Injury Management

6. A Review of Advances in Achilles Tendon Repair: Balancing Biomechanics and Biology

7. Wound Healing and Management

8. Hybrid Breast Reconstruction: Prepectoral Implant Combined with Lipofilling – Authors' Experience

9. A Plastic Surgeon's Perspective on the Management of Complicated Cases of Hidradenitis Suppurativa

The target audience comprises scholars and specialists in the field.

IntechOpen

Chapter 1

New Strategies for Prevention and Treatment of Sternal Wound Infection: Clinical Big Data-Driven Prediction and Precision Diagnosis-Treatment Integrated System in Plastic Surgery

Pan You, Jingjun Wei, Xin Zhou, Xiaohua Shi, Shuqing Huang, Dongli Fan and Zeyuan Lei

Abstract

This study focuses on developing novel strategies for preventing and treating sternal wound infection (SWI) by constructing a clinical big data-driven nomogram prediction model and exploring precision plastic surgery interventions. Retrospective analysis of 23,182 median sternotomy patients identified Body Mass Index (BMI), intensive care unit (ICU) stay, diabetes, and reoperation as the independent risk factors for SWI. The nomogram model demonstrated good discriminative ability (C–Statistic = 0.705) and clinical validity *via* ROC curve, calibration curve, and decision curve analyses. For treatment, 35 SWI patients were classified into superficial (SSWI) and deep (DSWI) infections: SSWI was managed with debridement, vacuum sealing drainage (VSD), and skin grafting, achieving a 92.6% cure rate, while DSWI utilized mixed reality (MR) technology for precise lesion localization combined with muscle flap transfer and foreign body-free wound closure, yielding a 100% cure rate with no recurrence during follow-up. The integrated approach of risk prediction and tailored plastic surgical strategies, enhanced by MR-guided precision, significantly improves SWI management and reduces recurrence, highlighting its clinical utility.

Keywords: sternal wound infection, risk factors, nomogram, prediction model, plastic surgery, repair and reconstruction, mixed reality technique

1. Introduction

Median sternotomy, due to high tension, hidden spaces, and numerous vital organs, is prone to postoperative (SWI), resulting in chronic refractory wounds that are difficult to control and repair. The incidence of SWI is 0.5–6% (12–20% in high-risk individuals), with a mortality rate of 14–47% and medical costs 2.8 times those of ordinary patients [1, 2]. Risk factors for SWI include patient-related factors (independent factors such as obesity, diabetes, and chronic obstructive pulmonary disease, COPD), and intraoperative/postoperative factors (e.g., operation duration, reoperation). Incidence varies by surgical type, with no consensus reached [3–5]. Treatment follows the principle of debridement: Mild cases require wound closure; severe cases need reconstruction with muscle flaps. Local antibiotics, VSD, and antibiotic use guided by drug sensitivity are also applicable [6, 7]. Preventive measures include preoperative skin preparation and disinfection, prophylactic antibiotics, perioperative glycemic control, and postoperative care [8]. Despite advancing technologies and improved preventive awareness among medical staff, the incidence of SWI has not significantly decreased, demanding urgent resolution. Next, the following will be elaborated on in two parts respectively.

2. Construction of a nomogram prediction model for sternal wound infection

Understanding the pathogenic characteristics and high-risk factors of SWI, and reducing its incidence and mortality through early detection, early intervention, and early treatment, is an urgent clinical problem to be solved. Kattan et al. first applied the nomogram in clinical practice to predict the postoperative recurrence of prostate cancer, with favorable outcomes [9]. Currently, the nomogram has become an excellent method for disease prediction, which can visualize the results of Logistic regression and quickly calculate the probability of event occurrence by summing up variable assignments [10].

However, there are currently no reports on nomograms related to SWI. The R programming language excels in statistical analysis and graphing, with advantages in data processing [11]. This study intends to use clinical data of SWI patients to analyze risk factors, construct a nomogram prediction model using R language, and verify its discriminative ability, calibration, and clinical validity. It aims to establish an efficient and accurate visual model, providing a tool for early clinical identification of high-risk patients to facilitate timely intervention.

2.1 Materials and methods

2.1.1 Clinical case information

The clinical data of this study were derived from the Second Affiliated Hospital of Army Medical University. A total of 23,182 patients who underwent median sternotomy in the Department of Cardiac Surgery from August 1, 2009 to July 31, 2019 were enrolled. They were divided into the observation group and the control group according to whether they developed SWI after surgery. The study was approved by the Ethics Committee of the hospital (Approval No.: 2019–Yan–No.037–01).

Inclusion criteria: aged ≥18 years; underwent median sternotomy; postoperative follow-up of at least 8 days. Exclusion criteria: aged <18 years; died within 8 days after surgery; missing or erroneous medical records data; immunodeficiency or positive HIV antibody. Patients in the observation group must meet the diagnostic criteria for SWI. Evaluation indicators included three categories: basic patient information (gender, age, BMI, etc.), surgical methods (heart valve replacement, congenital heart disease repair, etc.), and comorbidities (diabetes, hypertension, hyperlipidemia, etc.).

2.1.2 Statistical analysis

Univariate and multivariate logistic regression analyses were adopted. Normally distributed measurement data were expressed as mean ± standard deviation (mean ± SD) and analyzed by t-test; non-normally distributed measurement data were expressed as median (interquartile range) and analyzed by Wilcoxon rank-sum test; categorical data were expressed as frequency (%) and analyzed by chi-square test. Factors with statistical differences were screened by univariate Logistic regression. After collinearity diagnosis using Spearman correlation coefficient, factors without collinearity were included in multivariate Logistic regression to screen out independent risk factors for nomogram plotting.

Nomograms were plotted using the rms package in R language. The model was evaluated from three aspects: Discriminative ability was assessed by the area under the ROC curve and C-statistic (values>0.7 were considered valuable), which was plotted and calculated using the pROC package in R language; calibration was evaluated by calibration curves and Hosmer–Lemeshow test, with internal validation *via* 1000 Bootstrap samples; clinical validity was analyzed by decision curve analysis, plotted using the rmda package in R language. The test level was set at $\alpha = 0.05$, and $P < 0.05$ was considered statistically significant. Statistical analyses were performed using SPSS 25.0 (IBM, USA) and R software (R3.4.3, USA).

2.2 Results

2.2.1 Analysis of clinical indicators

A total of 15,426 patients were included in this study, among whom 5813 were male (37.7%) and 9613 were female (62.3%), with a male-to-female ratio of 0.6:1. Detailed clinical data are shown in **Table 1**. Among the types of thoracotomy, heart valve replacement surgery accounted for the largest number of cases (60.4%); the incidence of SWI after CABG was the highest, at 4.2%, as detailed in **Table 2**.

Hazards	All patients (n = 15,426)	Control group (n = 15,117)	Observation group (n = 309)
Age (years, median age)	48 (41–56)	48 (41–56)	51 (45–61)
Female [n (%)]	9613 (62.3)	9421 (62.3)	192 (62.1)
BMI ([kg/m^2], median BMI]	22.4 (20.2–24.7)	22.3 (20.2–24.6)	23.7 (21.8–26.3)
Obesity [(kg/m^2), (%)]	908 (5.9)	866 (5.7)	42 (13.6)
Surgical season [n (%)]			
Spring	5068 (32.9)	4962 (32.8)	106 (34.3)
Summer	3449 (22.4)	3370 (22.3)	79 (25.6)
Autumn	3415 (22.1)	3345 (22.1)	70 (22.7)
Winter	3494 (22.7)	3440 (22.8)	54 (17.5)
Intensive care unit time (days, median days)	1 (1–2)	1 (1–2)	2 (1–3)
Secondary surgery [n (%)]	135 (0.9)	119 (0.8)	16 (5.2)
Cardiogenic shock [n (%)]	22 (0.1)	20 (0.1)	2 (0.7)
Diabetes [n (%)]	636 (4.1)	598 (3.9)	38 (12.3)

Hazards	All patients (n = 15,426)	Control group (n = 15,117)	Observation group (n = 309)
Hypertension [n (%)]	1639 (10.6)	1572 (10.4)	67 (21.7)
Hyperlipidemia [n (%)]	418 (2.7)	400 (2.7)	18 (5.8)
Hypoproteinemia [n (%)]	150 (1.0)	142 (0.9)	8 (2.6)
COPD [n (%)]	132 (0.9)	129 (0.9)	3 (1.0)
Pulmonary hypertension [n (%)]	5419 (35.1)	5233 (34.6)	97 (31.4)
Renal failure [n (%)]	353 (2.3)	337 (2.2)	16 (5.2)
Hepatic failure [n (%)]	374 (2.4)	365 (2.4)	9 (2.9)
Cerebrovascular disease [n (%)]	789 (5.1)	771 (5.1)	18 (5.8)
Peripheral vascular disease [n (%)]	8 (0.1)	7 (0.1)	1 (0.3)
Respiratory infections [n (%)]	704 (4.6)	680 (4.5)	24 (7.8)
Atrial fibrillation [n (%)]	1823 (11.8)	1786 (11.8)	37 (12.0)
Myocardial infarction [n (%)]	241 (1.6)	229 (1.5)	12 (3.9)
Heart failure (New York classification ≥3) [n (%)]	9686 (62.8)	9484 (62.7)	202 (65.4)
Angina pectoris [n (%)]	937 (6.1)	891 (5.9)	46 (14.9)

Table 1.
General information of patients.

Type of thoracotomy	Examples and more the proportion of (%)	SWI sample size and probability of occurrence (%)
Heart valve replacement surgery	9315 (60.4)	175 (1.9)
Repair of congenital heart disease	2786 (18.1)	24 (0.9)
Coronary artery bypass grafting(CABG)	1426 (9.2)	60 (4.2)
Cardiac and vascular surgery	326 (2.1)	10 (3.1)
Heart tumor surgery	283 (1.8)	1 (0.4)
CABG + heart valve replacement	867 (5.6)	31 (3.6)
else	423 (2.7)	8 (1.9)

Table 2.
Clinical data of type of thoracotomy.

2.2.2 Results of univariate and multivariate logistic regression analyses

Univariate logistic regression identified 14 risk factors with statistical differences, including age, BMI, obesity, reoperation, intensive care unit stay, diabetes mellitus, hypertension, hyperlipidemia, hypoproteinemia, cardiogenic shock, renal failure, respiratory tract infection, myocardial infarction, and angina pectoris (see **Table 3** for details). Collinearity diagnosis (*via* Spearman correlation coefficient) showed no multicollinearity among these factors (see **Table 4** for details). Considering clinical significance and the need for nomogram construction, the above factors were incorporated into the multivariate logistic regression model using the enter method. Finally, BMI, intensive care unit stay, diabetes mellitus, and reoperation were confirmed as the independent predictive risk factors for SWI (see **Table 3** for details).

Project	Analysis of variance		Multiplicity	
	P price	OR (95% CI)	P price	OR (95% CI)
Age	0.000	1.030 (1.020–1.040)		
Female	0.947	0.992 (0.787–1.252)		
BMI	0.000	1.138 (1.104–1.173)	0.000	1.111 (1.075–1.147)
Fat	0.000	2.589 (1.856–3.610)		
Surgery season				
spring	ref.	ref.		
summer	0.536	1.097 (0.817–1.473)		
autumn	0.895	0.980 (0.722–1.329)		
winter	0.068	0.735 (0.528–1.023)		
ICU time	0.000	1.085 (1.065–1.105)	0.000	1.061 (1.038–1.085)
Secondary surgery	0.000	6.882 (4.033–11.746)	0.000	5.245 (2.930–9.391)
Cardiac shock	0.032	4.918 (1.144–21.131)		
Diabetes mellitus	0.000	3.404 (2.401–4.827)	0.005	1.764 (1.190–2.613)
Hypertension	0.000	2.386 (1.811–3.142)		
Hyperlipemia	0.001	2.276 (1.399–3.701)		
Hypoproteinemia	0.005	2.803 (1.363–5.766)		
COPD	0.824	1.139 (0.361–3.598)		
PAH	0.165	0.842 (0.661–1.073)		
Renal failure	0.001	2.395 (1.431–4.007)		
Hepatic failure	0.574	1.212 (0.620–2.372)		
Cerebrovascular disease	0.567	1.151 (0.711–1.863)		
Peripheral vascular disease	0.069	7.008 (0.860–57.136)		
Atrial fibrillation	0.931	1.015 (0.718–1.436)		
Myocardial infarction	0.001	2.627 (1.454–4.747)		
Heart failure (New York classification ≥3)	0.343	1.121 (0.885–1.421)		
Respiratory infection	0.007	1.788 (1.170–2.731)		
Angina pectoris	0.000	2.793 (2.027–3.848)		

Table 3.
Results of single factor and multi factor analysis of SWI.

Project	Tolerance	VIF
Age	0.829	1.206
BMI	0.904	1.106
ICU time	0.873	1.145
Secondary surgery	0.987	1.022
Cardiac shock	0.982	1.018
Diabetes mellitus	0.898	1.114
Hypertension	0.792	1.262
Hyperlipemia	0.955	1.047
Hypoproteinemia	0.970	1.031
Renal failure	0.937	1.067
Respiratory infection	0.940	1.063
Myocardial infarction	0.936	1.069
Angina pectoris	0.813	1.231

Table 4.
Co-linearity diagnostic results.

2.2.3 Construction of the prediction model and presentation of the nomogram

The above results indicated that the independent risk factors for SWI were BMI, intensive care unit (ICU) stay, diabetes mellitus, and reoperation. Based on these, a prediction model was constructed and a nomogram was plotted (**Figure 1**). Instructions for using the nomogram: BMI (kg/m^2) and ICU stay (days) are quantitative variables; reoperation and diabetes mellitus are qualitative variables categorized

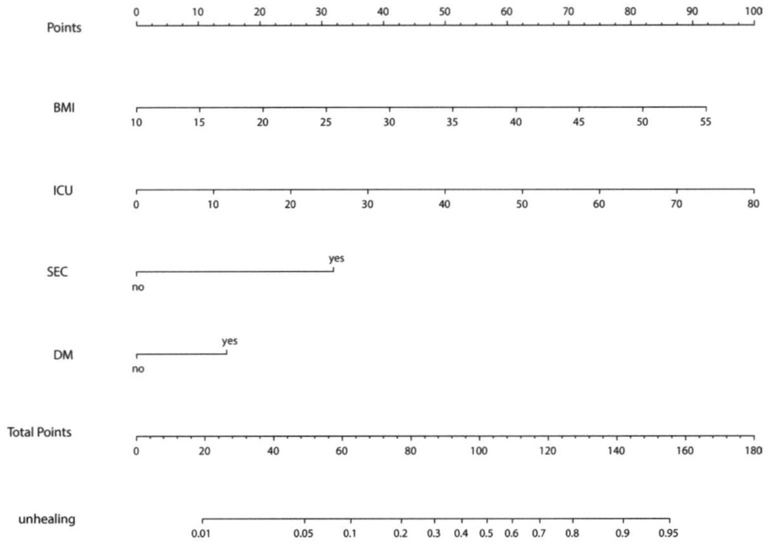

Figure 1.
Nomogram for predicting SWI.

as "yes" or "no." Each factor corresponds to the "Score" axis to obtain the respective score; the sum of these scores corresponds to the "Total Score" axis, which gives the probability of SWI occurrence.

2.2.4 Evaluation results of discriminative ability, calibration, and validity of the nomogram prediction model

Discriminative ability: The area under the ROC curve (C-statistic) of the model was 0.705 (95%CI: 0.646–0.803), indicating the model is effective. The optimal cut-off value of 0.018 corresponded to a sensitivity of 0.702 and a specificity of 0.739, further verifying the reliability of the model. See **Figure 2**.

Calibration: Calibration curve analysis showed that the calibration curve of the model's predicted probability and actual probability was close to the ideal curve, showing good consistency. In the Hosmer–Lemeshow goodness-of-fit test, the χ^2 value was 6.987 and $P = 0.538$ ($P > 0.05$), indicating that the model had good goodness-of-fit and high predictive performance. See **Figure 3**.

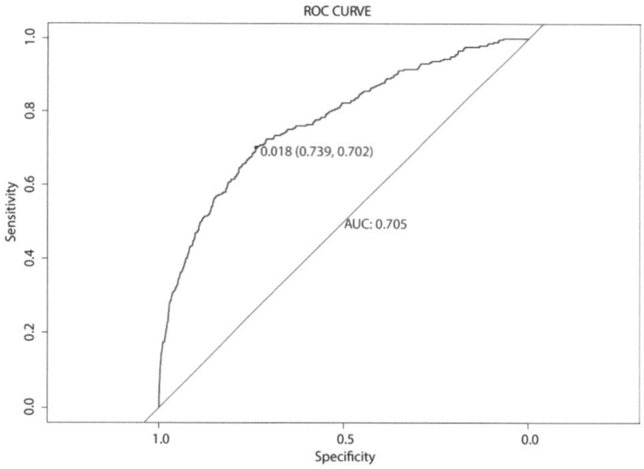

Figure 2.
ROC curve of the SWI prediction model.

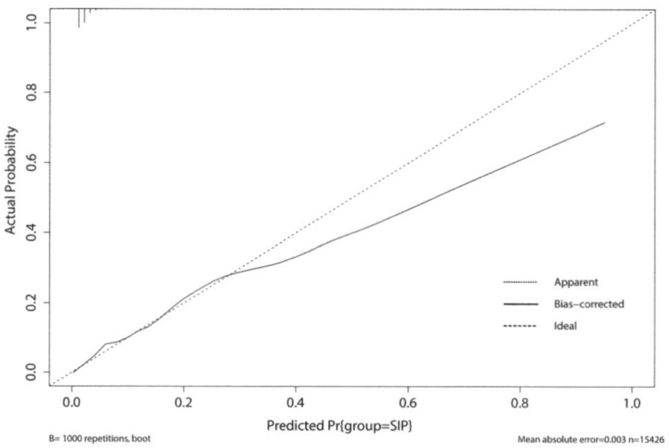

Figure 3.
Calibration curve of the SWI prediction model.

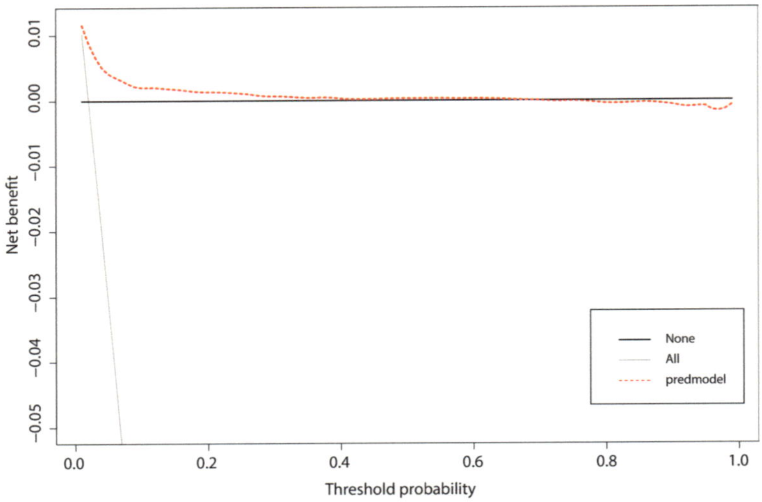

Figure 4.
Decision curve of the SWI prediction model.

Validity: The clinical decision curve showed that when the SWI cut-off value was 0.018, the net benefit was >0, and the net benefit rate within the cut-off range was all >0, indicating that the model has good clinical validity. See **Figure 4**.

2.3 Discussion

Due to its special location, median sternotomy has a relatively high risk of SWI [12]. Among thoracotomies in cardiovascular surgery, SWI is most common after CABG and combined surgeries, and CABG accounts for the largest proportion of patients who progress to DSWI postoperatively [13]. In this study, the incidence of SWI after CABG was 4.2%, and 3.6% after combined surgeries. In contrast, heart valve replacement surgery, which accounted for 60.4% of cases (9315 cases), had an SWI incidence of 1.9% (175 cases). Additionally, the use of bilateral internal thoracic arteries in CABG and prolonged operation time are the independent risk factors for SWI.

In this study, diabetic patients accounted for 12.3% in the observation group, significantly higher than 4.0% in the control group. Poor glycemic control is an important risk factor for SWI, so perioperative glycemic control is necessary. Furnary et al. also confirmed that glycemic control can reduce SWI, and postoperative stress can also affect healing [14]. The incidence of SWI in patients with reoperation was 5.5 times that in the control group, and re-exploration under non-sterile conditions is an independent risk factor [15].

Obesity is associated with SWI, as it can cause local ischemia; prolonged ICU stay increases the risk of SWI [16, 17]. The existing Gatti assessment scale is only applicable to post-CABG patients [12], while the prediction model in this study has a wider application range and is easy to operate. However, this study is a single-center retrospective study, requiring multi-center and external validation. In conclusion, this model can promote multidisciplinary collaboration, and the next step is to establish a more comprehensive wound early warning and intervention model.

3. Plastic surgery diagnosis and treatment strategies for sternal wound infection

The occurrence of SWI poses significant challenges to clinical practice. Due to insufficient attention, lack of unified diagnosis and treatment protocols, and its delayed onset, many patients are diagnosed only after discharge, missing the optimal treatment window. In particular, complex DSWI increases mortality with severe consequences. Therefore, it is crucial to determine the scope and layers of infection through appropriate early examinations and formulate a reasonable plan. Although extensive research has been conducted on the risk factors of SWI, there is no unified diagnosis and treatment protocol. The traditional approach of regular debridement combined with repeated dressing changes is inefficient, time-consuming, and costly. This study aims to improve the process through accurate diagnosis and classified treatment (using VSD, muscle flap transfer, etc.). In addition, DSWI involves multiple layers of infection, and difficulty in accurate preoperative localization leads to incomplete debridement and postoperative recurrence. However, MR technology can process medical image data and provide auxiliary diagnostic and therapeutic tools through 3D visualization [18]. It is intended to be used for preoperative localization of infection scope, guiding intraoperative debridement to ensure thoroughness, reducing recurrence, and assisting in doctor-patient communication and postoperative follow-up.

3.1 Materials and methods

3.1.1 Clinical data

Clinical data of 35 patients with SWI in the Department of Plastic Surgery from March 2017 to March 2019 were collected. The time from the occurrence of SWI after cardiac surgery to medical consultation ranged from 7 to 1460 days, among which 25 cases (71.4%) had a duration >30 days. All patients had wounds or sinuses at the sternal incision, with areas ranging from $0.5 \times 1.0\ cm^2$ to $3.0 \times 12.0\ cm^2$. Wound secretion culture was positive in 10 cases. This study was approved by the Ethics Committee of the Second Affiliated Hospital of Army Medical University (Approval No.: 2019–Yan–No.037–01). Other information is shown in **Table 5**.

3.1.2 Methods

Based on the severity of patients' conditions, accurate diagnosis was made, and personalized treatment plans were formulated by classification. SSWI was mainly treated with debridement, VSD, skin grafting, etc. For DSWI, MR technology was used to assist in accurately locating lesions, and plastic surgery repair and reconstruction techniques such as muscle flap transfer and foreign-body-free wound plasty were adopted. Clinical efficacy was evaluated according to SWI wound recovery, hospital stay, follow-up status, cure rate, etc.

3.1.2.1 Basic treatment methods

After admission, SWI patients first received a comprehensive assessment of their condition, active treatment of primary diseases, and maintenance of stable blood glucose and electrolyte balance. Examinations including chest CT, electrocardiogram (ECG), echocardiography, blood routine, heart failure markers, procalcitonin (PCT),

Project	SWI(n = 35)	SSWI(n = 27)	DSWI(n = 8)
Age (median age)	17 ~ 71 (50)	17 ~ 69 (49)	52 ~ 71 (63)
Female [case (%)]	27 (77.1)	21 (77.8)	6 (75.0)
BMI > 24 kg/m^2 [case (%)]	20 (57.1)	17 (63.0)	3 (37.5)
Originated from rural areas [case (%)]	21 (60.0)	16 (59.3)	5 (62.5)
Comorbid underlying diseases [case (%)]			
Hypertension	6 (17.1)	4 (14.8)	2 (25.0)
Diabetes mellitus	7 (20.0)	3 (11.1)	4 (50.0)
Cardiac insufficiency	3 (8.6)	2 (7.4)	1 (12.5)
Primary heart diseases [case (%)]			
Rheumatic heart disease	26 (70.2)	19 (70.3)	7 (87.5)
Congenital heart disease	3 (8.6)	3 (11.1)	0 (0.0)
Aortic dissection	3 (8.6)	3 (11.1)	0 (0.0)
Coronary heart disease	2 (5.7)	1 (3.7)	1 (12.5)

Table 5.
Basic clinical data of patients.

hepatic and renal functions, and wound secretion culture + drug sensitivity test were completed. Sensitive antibiotics were administered when necessary, and coagulation function was closely monitored.

3.1.2.2 Treatment of SSWI

Debridement and VSD were sequentially used according to the condition, and skin grafting was performed to cover residual wounds if necessary. For SWI debridement, foreign bodies and infected necrotic tissues (such as sutures, infected skin, and soft tissues) must be completely removed; the incision was irrigated starting from the most contaminated center to the surrounding area. VSD application protocols: For SSWI patients with clean and dry incisions, intermittent negative pressure mode (60–80 mmHg) was selected to promote circulation; for those with severe infection and excessive secretions, continuous negative pressure mode (80–120 mmHg) was used for timely fluid drainage. The device was replaced every 5–10 days, and the frequency of use depended on drainage fluid, wound recovery, and the patient's condition. For some patients, residual incisions could be directly sutured after VSD, and sutures were removed postoperatively according to recovery. When the area of residual incisions was large, an appropriate donor site could be selected for skin grafting, which could be performed multiple times.

3.1.2.3 Treatment of DSWI

Repair and reconstruction were performed using muscle flap transfer and foreign-body-free wound plasty. All patients underwent 64-slice chest spiral CT scanning preoperatively (slice thickness < 1 mm). Image data were stored in Digital Imaging and Communications in Medicine (DICOM) format, processed by contrast-enhanced multi-detector CT, and then, 3D reconstruction of multiple sites such as ribs and costal cartilages was performed using Mimics software (Materiaise's Interactive

Medical Image Control System). After programmed segmentation and registration, they were integrated into a 3D mesh model in STL format (stereolithography), with each tissue structure marked in different colors. The model allows 360° rotation and scaling, facilitating multi-dimensional observation of the infected area and adjacent parts. Subsequently, a 3D stereoscopic reconstruction model was constructed via 3D hyper-rendering technology. After processing such as function setting and parameter adjustment, it was applied to MR equipment, thereby achieving smooth doctor-patient communication, rational preoperative planning, and precise intraoperative guidance (see **Figure 5** for the implementation process of MR technology and **Figure 6** for application examples).

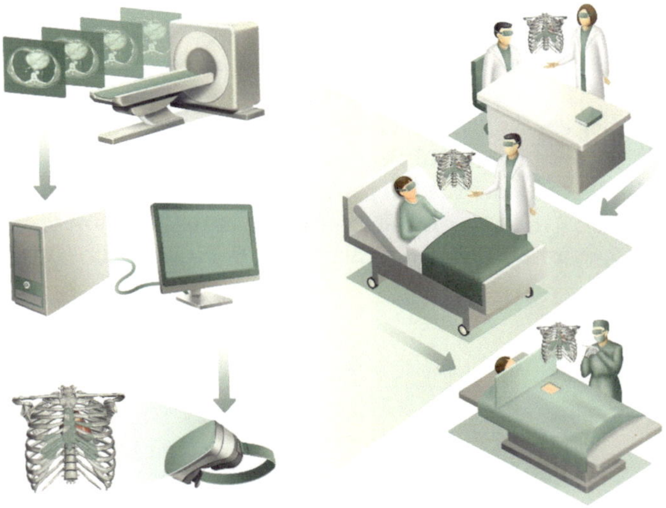

Figure 5.
Implementation steps of MR technology in DSWI diagnosis and treatment.

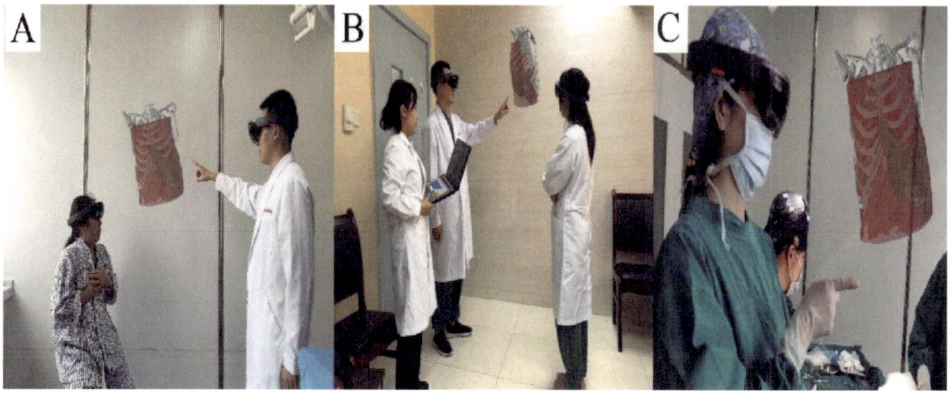

Figure 6.
Application examples of MR technology in DSWI diagnosis and treatment. A: Doctor-patient communication; B: preoperative planning; C: intraoperative guidance.

After accurate localization of the infected lesion, surgical debridement and repair-reconstruction are required. Under general anesthesia, the original sternal incision is extended by 1 cm to resect necrotic tissues and scars, followed by thorough layer-by-layer debridement. Based on MR technology localization, infected sternum, costal cartilages, soft tissues, and foreign bodies (such as sutures, steel wires, bone wax) are removed. The wound is alternately irrigated with hydrogen peroxide solution and normal saline, and contaminated instruments are replaced. Reconstruction plans are designed according to the lesion location. Taking pectoralis major muscle flap transfer as an example: Subcutaneous tissue is dissected along the superficial layer of the pectoralis major fascia on one side of the original incision, with layer-by-layer dissection and hemostasis. The lateral part of the pectoralis major is transected according to the defect size and inverted inward, and its deep surface is dissected to form a muscle flap, which is then filled into the defect area. The nutrient vascular pedicle 1.5 cm beside the sternum must be preserved. Hemostasis is achieved at the donor site, and a drainage tube is placed (removed when the drainage volume is <15 mL/24 h). Foreign-body-free wound plasty is used to fix the muscle flap and close the incision: 7–0 suture is used to fix the muscle flap through the full thickness of subcutaneous tissue and skin, with knots tied outside the contralateral skin edge; gauze is placed under the knots to reduce tension. Sutures are removed about 10 days postoperatively according to healing status. Relevant operations are shown in **Figure 7** (pectoralis major muscle flap) and **Figure 8** (foreign-body-free plasty).

3.2 Results

3.2.1 Efficacy analysis

For 27 patients with SSWI, the average in-hospital treatment time was 57 days (range 5–126 days), with a cure rate of 92.6%. VSD was replaced three times on average. Among them, 25 cases achieved primary intention healing of the incision, and 2 cases were discharged without cure. For 8 patients with DSWI, the average

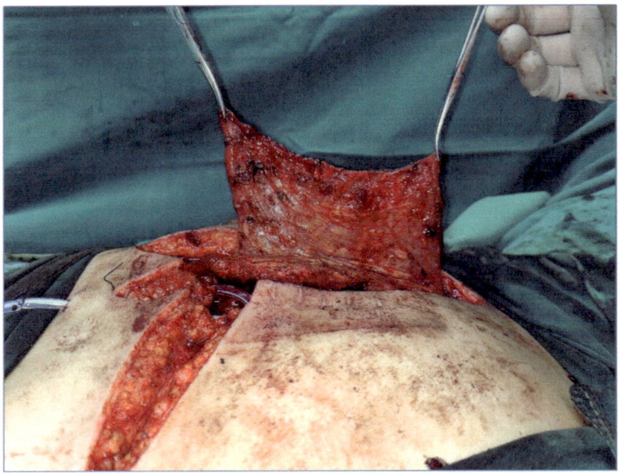

Figure 7.
Pectoralis major muscle flap.

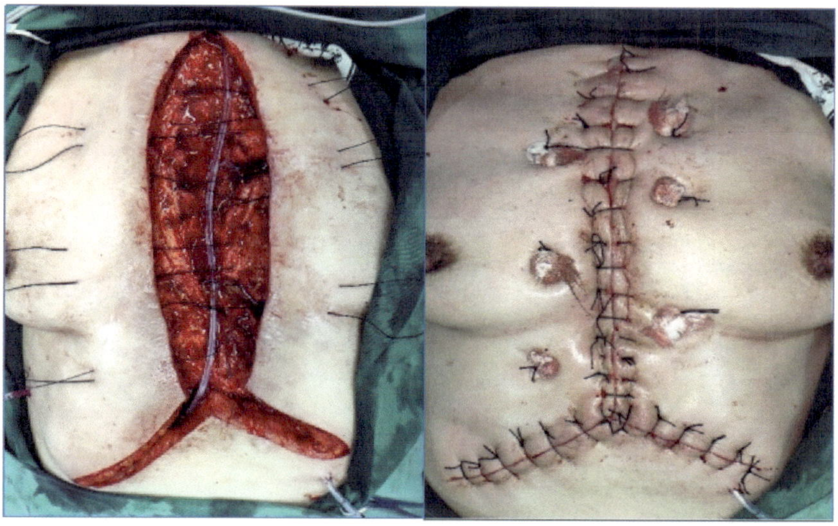

Figure 8.
Foreign-body–free wound plasty.

in-hospital treatment time was 32 days (range 10–96 days), with a cure rate of 100%. All of them underwent accurate lesion localization using MR technology, and were treated with different types of muscle flap transfer and foreign-body-free wound plasty. Among them, seven cases achieved primary intention healing of the incision, and one case achieved subcrustal healing. The function of the muscle flap donor site was not affected, and no recurrence was observed during the 2-month to 2-year follow-up.

3.2.2 Typical cases

3.2.2.1 Case 1

A 48-year-old female patient developed SSWI 20 days after valve replacement for rheumatic heart disease. Physical examination showed a chest median wound of approximately 203 cm^2, 1 cm deep, involving the full-length skin and subcutaneous soft tissue of the sternum. Wound secretion culture was positive for *Staphylococcus aureus*. The patient's basic condition was good without special complications. Conservative treatment with debridement combined with VSD was adopted. After 2 uses of VSD, the wound shrank and improved, so the residual wound was directly sutured. After three dressing changes, primary intention healing was achieved 9 days postoperatively, and the sutures were removed before discharge. During the 3-month follow-up, there was no recurrence. The diagnosis, treatment, and follow-up process are detailed in **Figure 9**.

3.2.2.2 Case 2

A 60-year-old male patient underwent median sternotomy for mediastinal tumor resection 4 months ago. The scar ulcerated and became infected 3 months ago, and he was admitted to the Department of Plastic Surgery. Physical examination:

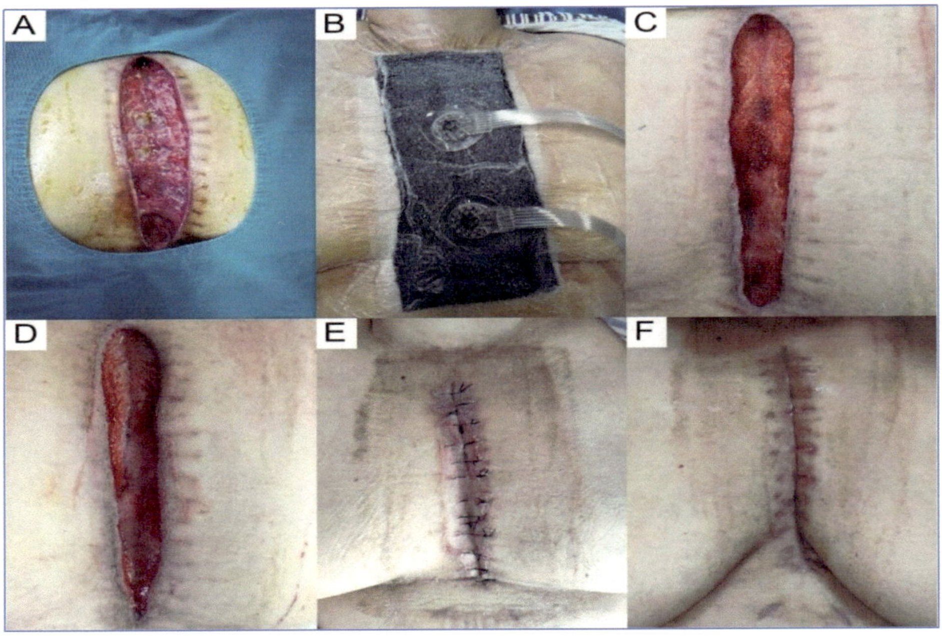

Figure 9.
Diagnosis, treatment, and follow-up process of Case 1. A: 20 days after valve replacement; B: VSD application status; C: after first VSD; D: after second VSD; E: after direct suture; F: wound healing at discharge.

A postoperative scar approximately 30 cm in length was present in the midline of the sternum, with a wound at the xiphoid process. The wound had a diameter of 2 cm, with white viscous secretions on the surface, and mild redness and swelling of the surrounding skin. Wound exudate culture indicated Aspergillus infection. Combined with chest CT reconstructed by MR technology, the diagnosis was DSWI, involving the middle and lower sternum, multiple bilateral costal cartilages, and intercostal soft tissues. Treatment began with thorough debridement. Due to extensive tissue defects, reconstruction was performed using pectoralis major muscle flap combined with rectus abdominis muscle flap transplantation. Postoperatively, voriconazole capsules and glutathione tablets were administered for symptomatic treatment. The incision achieved primary intention healing and sutures were removed. Follow-up for half a year showed no recurrence, and the limb function at the muscle flap donor site was normal. The diagnosis, treatment and follow-up process are detailed in **Figure 10**.

3.2.2.3 Case 3

A 57-year-old female patient developed SWI over 1 month after valve replacement for rheumatic heart disease and was admitted to the Department of Plastic Surgery. On admission, a 42 cm^2 wound was found at the lower sternum, 2 cm deep, with red and swollen wound edges, marked tenderness, and yellowish-white viscous fluid upon squeezing. Wound secretion culture was negative. Combined with chest CT reconstructed by mixed reality technology, the diagnosis was DSWI. The patient had a 4-year history of diabetes mellitus, and MR showed that the infection involved the middle and lower sternum, bilateral 3rd–4th intercostal soft tissues, and 4th–7th costal cartilages. Thorough debridement of the infected

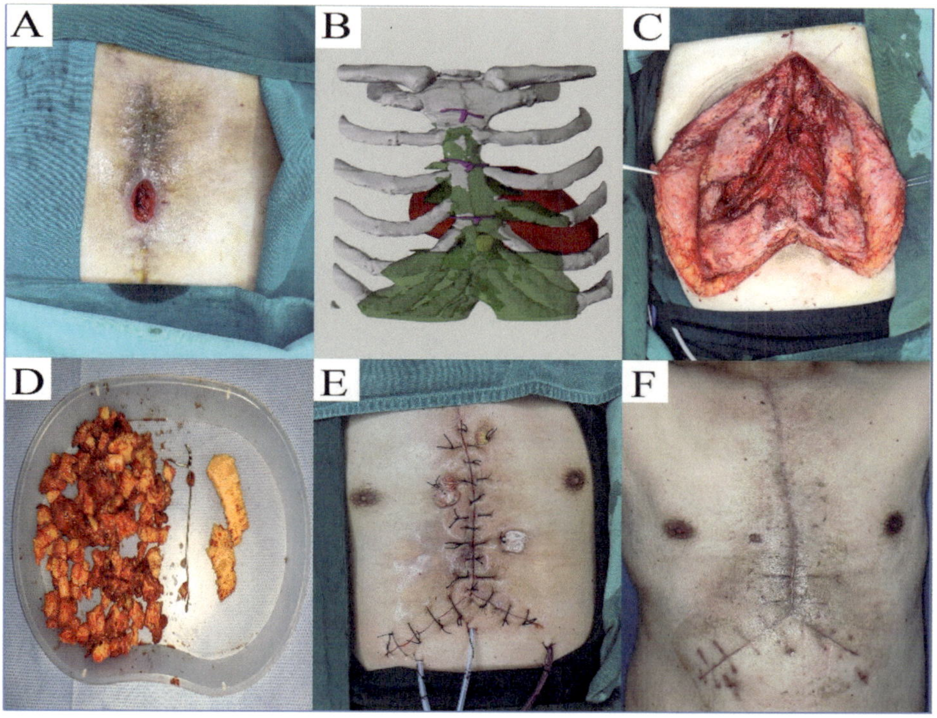

Figure 10.
Diagnosis, treatment, and follow-up process of Case 2. A: Over 4 months after mediastinal tumor surgery; B: preoperative localization of infected area by MR technology (shadow area); C: wound after thorough debridement; D: removed infected tissues (sternum, costal cartilage, soft tissue) and foreign bodies (sutures, steel wires); E: immediate postoperative period; F: 2 months after operation.

lesion and pectoralis major muscle flap transfer were performed for repair. The incision achieved primary intention healing postoperatively, with normal limb movement at the muscle flap donor site, and no recurrence was observed during the 3-month follow-up. The diagnosis, treatment, and follow-up process are detailed in **Figure 11**.

3.3 Discussion

SWI is characterized by a long course of disease and high costs. Some patients have insidious onset, which may easily lead to delayed treatment and increased mortality. Therefore, early accurate diagnosis and a reasonable diagnosis and treatment plan are crucial. Most patients develop symptoms such as low-grade fever within 1 month after surgery, but some with insidious onset are prone to delayed treatment. Treatment mainly includes antibiotics and thorough debridement. With the improvement in the application of muscle flaps, the effect of treating DSWI is significant. Therefore, after confirmation, classified diagnosis and treatment should be performed, and thorough debridement should be conducted as early as possible to prevent SSWI from progressing to DSWI [19]. VSD is the main treatment for SSWI, and skin grafting is the preferred option for superficial wounds. Early thorough debridement is an ideal strategy for DSWI [20]. However, previous debridement relied on visual experience, which was prone to misjudgment. Accurate localization of infected foci is the key. Traditional imaging has poor or limited ability to identify early changes of DSWI,

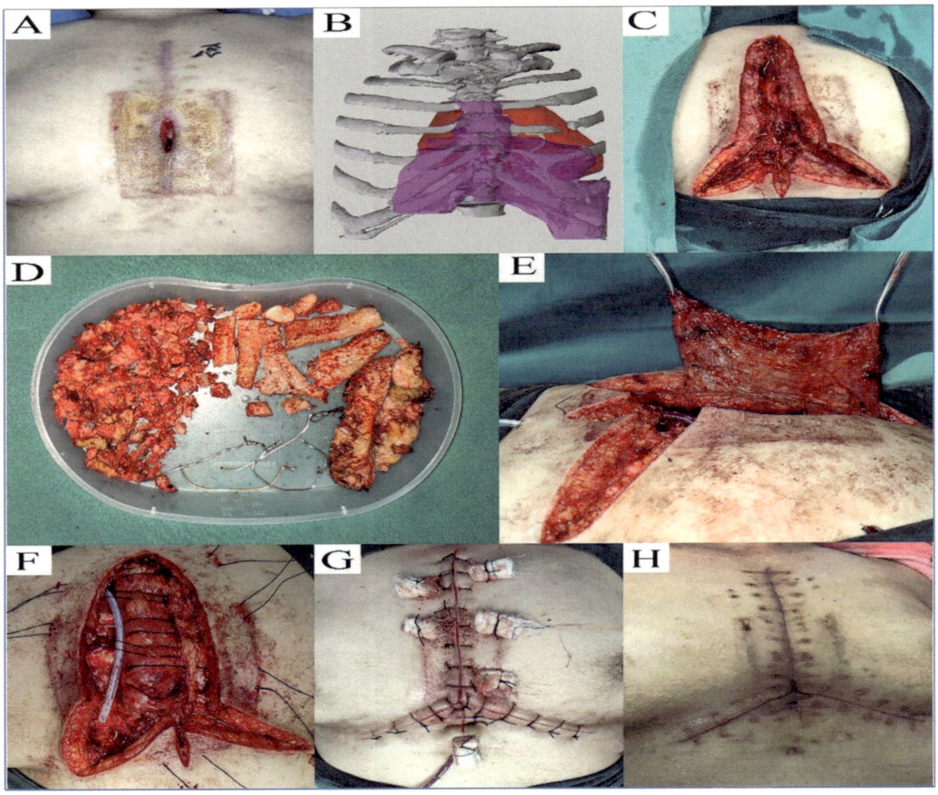

Figure 11.
Diagnosis, treatment, and follow-up process of Case 3. A: Over 1 month after valve replacement; B: preoperative localization of infected area by MR technology (shadow area); C: wound after thorough debridement; D: removed infected tissues (sternum, costal cartilage, soft tissue) and foreign bodies (sutures, steel wires); E: dissected pectoralis major muscle flap; F: incision closure by foreign-body-free wound plasty; G: immediate postoperative period; H: 2 weeks after operation.

while MR technology can detect tiny lesions, guide debridement, and improve efficiency. It converts 2D images into 3D visualized structures, facilitating doctor-patient communication to reduce disputes [21]. Currently, it is widely used in surgical design and other fields, which can improve surgical intelligence and medical quality.

4. Conclusion

SWI tends to progress to chronic refractory wounds; clinically, efforts should focus on reducing its incidence and improving cure rates. Large-sample analysis identified BMI, ICU stay, reoperation, and diabetes as the independent risk factors. The R-language nomogram model exhibits strong performance, aiding its adoption for early intervention. A stratified treatment approach was employed: SSWI centers on debridement and VSD; DSWI utilizes MR for precise localization to aid diagnosis/management, coupled with reconstructive techniques like muscle flap transfer. Both yielded favorable outcomes, with MR notably ensuring thorough debridement to lower recurrence. Future studies should enhance interdisciplinary collaboration, refine early warning/intervention protocols, and optimize diagnostic/therapeutic workflows.

Author details

Pan You[1*], Jingjun Wei[2], Xin Zhou[3], Xiaohua Shi[1], Shuqing Huang[1], Dongli Fan[1] and Zeyuan Lei[1]

1 Department of Plastic and Cosmetic Surgery, Second Affiliated Hospital of Army Medical University, Chongqing, China

2 Chongqing Institute of Foreign Studies, Chongqing, China

3 Jinfeng Laboratory, Chongqing, China

*Address all correspondence to: youpanzhengxing@163.com

References

[1] Franco S, Herrera AM, Atehortua M, et al. Use of steel bands in sternotomy closure: Implications in high-risk cardiac surgical population [J]. Interactive Cardiovascular and Thoracic Surgery. 2009;**8**(2):200-205. DOI: 10.1510/icvts.2008.188136

[2] Sajja LR, Mannam G, Dandu SB, et al. Reduction of sternal wound infections in diabetic patients undergoing off-pump coronary artery bypass surgery and using modified pedicle bilateral internal thoracic artery harvest technique [J]. The Journal of Thoracic and Cardiovascular Surgery. 2012;**144**(2):480-485. DOI: 10.1016/j.jtcvs.2012.03.024

[3] Lu JC, Grayson AD, Jha P, et al. Risk factors for sternal wound infection and mid-term survival following coronary artery bypass surgery [J]. European Journal of Cardio-Thoracic Surgery. 2003;**23**(6):943-949. DOI: 10.1016/s1010-7940(03)00137-4

[4] Meszaros K, Fuehrer U, Grogg S, et al. Risk factors for sternal wound infection after open heart operations vary according to type of operation [J]. The Annals of Thoracic Surgery. 2016;**101**(4):1418-1425. DOI: 10.1016/j.athoracsur.2015.09.010

[5] Lemaignen A, Birgand G, Ghodhbane W, et al. Sternal wound infection after cardiac surgery: Incidence and risk factors according to clinical presentation [J]. Clinical Microbiology and Infection. 2015;**21**(7):674 e11-8. DOI: 10.1016/j.cmi.2015.03.025

[6] Ridderstolpe L, Gill H, Granfeldt H, et al. Superficial and deep sternal wound complications: Incidence, risk factors and mortality [J]. European Journal of Cardio-Thoracic Surgery. 2001;**20**(6):1168-1175. DOI: 10.1016/s1010-7940(01)00991-5

[7] Engelman R, Shahian D, Shemin R, et al. The Society of Thoracic Surgeons practice guideline series: Antibiotic prophylaxis in cardiac surgery, part II: Antibiotic choice [J]. The Annals of Thoracic Surgery. 2007;**83**(4):1569-1576. DOI: 10.1016/j.athoracsur.2006.09.046

[8] Yusuf E, Chan M, Renz N, et al. Current perspectives on diagnosis and management of sternal wound infections [J]. Infection and Drug Resistance. 2018;**11**:961-968. DOI: 10.2147/IDR.S130172

[9] Kattan MW. Nomograms are superior to staging and risk grouping systems for identifying high-risk patients: Preoperative application in prostate cancer [J]. Current Opinion in Urology. 2003;**13**(2):111-116. DOI: 10.1097/00042307-200303000-00005

[10] Iasonos A, Schrag D, Raj GV, et al. How to build and interpret a nomogram for cancer prognosis [J]. Journal of Clinical Oncology. 2008;**26**(8):1364-1370. DOI: 10.1200/JCO.2007.12.9791

[11] Arai H. A function for the R programming language to recast garnet analyses into end-members: Revision and porting of Muhling and Griffin's method [J]. Computers & Geosciences. 2010;**36**(3):406-409. DOI: 10.1016/j.cageo.2009.05.007

[12] Gatti G, Barbati G, Luzzati R, et al. Prospective validation of a predictive scoring system for deep sternal wound infection after routine bilateral internal thoracic artery grafting [J]. Interactive

Cardiovascular and Thoracic Surgery. 2016;**22**(5):606-611. DOI: 10.1093/icvts/ivw016

[13] Sharif M, Wong CHM, Harky A. Sternal wound infections, risk factors and management - How far are we? A literature review [J]. Heart, Lung & Circulation. 2019;**28**(6):835-843. DOI: 10.1016/j.hlc.2019.01.008

[14] Furnary AP, Zerr KJ, Grunkemeier GL, et al. Continuous intravenous insulin infusion reduces the incidence of deep sternal wound infection in diabetic patients after cardiac surgical procedures [J]. The Annals of Thoracic Surgery. 1999;**67**(2):352-360; discussion 60-62. DOI: 10.1016/s0003-4975(99)00014-4

[15] Munoz P, Menasalvas A, Bernaldo de Quiros JC, et al. Postsurgical mediastinitis: A case-control study [J]. Clinical Infectious Diseases. 1997;**25**(5):1060-1064. DOI: 10.1086/516068

[16] Khan T, Muise ES, Iyengar P, et al. Metabolic dysregulation and adipose tissue fibrosis: Role of collagen VI [J]. Molecular and Cellular Biology. 2009;**29**(6):1575-1591. DOI: 10.1128/MCB.01300-08

[17] Buja A, Zampieron A, Cavalet S, et al. An update review on risk factors and scales for prediction of deep sternal wound infections [J]. International Wound Journal. 2012;**9**(4):372-386. DOI: 10.1111/j.1742-481X.2011.00896.x

[18] Chen AD, Lin SJ. Discussion: Mixed reality with HoloLens: Where virtual reality meets augmented reality in the operating room [J]. Plastic and Reconstructive Surgery. 2017;**140**(5):1071-1072. DOI: 10.1097/PRS.0000000000003817

[19] Kamel GN, Jacobson J, Rizzo AM, et al. Analysis of immediate versus delayed sternal reconstruction with pectoralis major advancement versus turnover muscle flaps [J]. Journal of Reconstructive Microsurgery. 2019;**35**(8):602-608. DOI: 10.1055/s-0039-1688760

[20] Berdajs DA, Trampuz A, Ferrari E, et al. Delayed primary versus late secondary wound closure in the treatment of postsurgical sternum osteomyelitis [J]. Interactive Cardiovascular and Thoracic Surgery. 2011;**12**(6):914-918. DOI: 10.1510/icvts.2010.263483

[21] Ke F, Lee S, Xu X. Teaching training in a mixed - reality reality integrated reality reality reality integrated learning environment [J]. Computers in Human Behavior. 2016;**62**:212-220. DOI: 10.1016/j.chb.2016.03.094

Chapter 2

Evolution and Innovation in Reconstructive Breast Surgery: A Comprehensive Review

Alba Mayra Padilla, Celina Verónica Kishi, Heriberto Contreras, Karla Elizabeth Rincón, Pablo Meneses and Maximiliano Sánchez

Abstract

This chapter provides a comprehensive overview of contemporary techniques and recent advances in reconstructive breast surgery, integrating evidence-based practices, surgical outcomes, and patient-centered considerations. Both autologous and implant-based reconstruction methods are examined in detail, with emphasis on indications, risks, and comparative outcomes. Particular attention is given to the timing of reconstruction in the setting of postmastectomy radiation therapy (PMRT), the role of acellular dermal matrices (ADMs), and the impact of comorbidities such as diabetes mellitus on complication rates. Recent meta-analyses and multicenter studies indicate that autologous reconstruction—particularly with deep inferior epigastric perforator (DIEP) flaps—offers greater patient satisfaction and lower long-term complication rates compared to implant-based techniques, although with increases operative complexity and donor-site morbidity. Evidence suggests that microvascular breast reconstruction can be safely performed as early as 6 months after the completion of PMRT, without a significant increase in major complications. Furthermore, key predictors of postoperative complications, including obesity, hypertension, and diabetes, are identified to support preoperative risk stratification and optimization. Overall, the chapter underscores the importance of individualized surgical planning, multidisciplinary collaboration, and long-term follow-up in achieving optimal outcomes for patients undergoing breast reconstruction after cancer treatment.

Keywords: breast surgery, autologous reconstruction, postmastectomy reconstruction, microvascular reconstruction, implant-based reconstruction, preoperative optimization, breast review

1. Introduction

Breast cancer is the most frequently diagnosed malignancy among women globally, with an estimated 2.3 million new cases and 685,000 deaths reported in 2020 alone [1]. Its burden is projected to increase dramatically, with incidence expected to rise by 38% and mortality by 68% by the year 2050 [2]. While advances in oncology therapies have significantly improved survival, survivorship issues such as body image, psychological work being and sexual health have gained increasing attention. In this context, breast reconstruction has emerged as a vital component of comprehensive breast cancer care. Beyond restoring physical contour, reconstruction contributes to emotional healing, improves quality of life and supports reintegration to daily social activities [3, 4]. The use of validated instruments such as the BREAST-Q has reinforced the positive psychological impact of reconstructive procedures, particularly in patients undergoing immediate or autologous reconstruction [5].

The evolution of breast reconstruction techniques reflects broader advances in plastic surgery and microsurgical innovation. Early attempts date back to the 1800s with a transplant of a lipoma to a mastectomy site [6]. Implant-based breast reconstruction, according to Spear and Onyewy, is staged reconstruction using tissue expanders and implants that can be safely performed even in previously irradiated patients, although complication rates tend to be higher compared to non-irradiated cases [7]. Recent meta-analyses have shown that prepectoral implant placement offers comparable safety to subpectoral reconstruction, with significantly lower rates of animation deformity and postoperative pain, while prepectoral approaches tend to show high rates of seroma and visible rippling [8].

Subsequent decades witnessed the development of musculocutaneous flaps, particularly the transverse rectus abdominis myocutaneous (TRAM) flap and its evolution into the muscle-sparing TRAM and deep inferior epigastric perforator (DIEP) flap, which preserve abdominal function while offering superior esthetic outcomes [9, 10]. More recently, refinements in microsurgical technique including the use of alternative perforator flaps and improved recipient vessel selection have enhanced success rates and aesthetic outcomes in autologous reconstruction [11]. Preoperative imaging, such as high- resolution CT angiography (CTA) and ultrasound, now plays a central role in perforator mapping, reducing operative time and improving flap reliability [12, 13]. Meanwhile, nerve coaptation (neurotization) techniques have demonstrated significantly improved sensory recovery compared to non-innervated DIEP flaps [14]. Finally, enhanced recovery after surgery (ERAS) protocols have been shown to reduce opioid consumption and hospital length of stay after autologous reconstruction without increasing complication rates [15].

This chapter provides a comprehensive review of breast reconstruction, tracing its historical evolution and highlighting current practices and innovations. We will explore both implant-based and autologous techniques, patient selection criteria, timing, outcomes and complication management. The objective is to offer a multidisciplinary evidence-based framework of contemporary and future practice in reconstructive breast surgery.

2. Classification of reconstructive techniques

Breast reconstruction following mastectomy has evolved into a multifaceted field that encompasses a broad range of surgical approaches, each tailored to address patient-specific anatomical, oncologic, and psychosocial considerations. The classification of reconstructive techniques is not merely a matter of academic organization; it is fundamental to clinical decision-making and surgical planning.

Reconstruction can be broadly categorized by the type of tissue used, autologous versus implant-based, as well as by the timing of the procedure (immediate, delayed, or delayed-immediate), and whether it is performed in one or two stages. These categories are not mutually exclusive; rather, they offer a structured framework to help clinicians navigate increasingly complex reconstructive options in the era of multimodal cancer treatment and patient-centered care [16, 17].

Implant-based reconstruction remains the most commonly performed approach worldwide due to its relative simplicity and shorter operative time [18]. However, autologous tissue reconstruction (particularly with perforator flaps such as the DIEP) has shown superior long-term outcomes in selected patients, especially those with a history of postmastectomy radiotherapy (PMRT) or contraindications to implants [19, 20]. Recent evidence underscores the importance of selecting techniques not only on surgical feasibility, but also based on patient-reported satisfaction, complications profiles, and functional outcomes [21].

The incorporation of newer modalities, such as prepectoral implant placement and the use of acellular dermal matrices (ADMs), has further diversified available options, particularly in settings where preservation of the pectoralis major muscle is desired [22–24]. Simultaneously, delayed and delayed-immediate strategies remain valuable for patients requiring postoperative radiotherapy, allowing for better management of irradiated tissue beds and minimizing reconstructive failure risk [25, 26].

Understanding the classification of these reconstructive modalities is essential for ensuring the highest standard of care and aligning surgical choices with both evidence-based protocols and patient goals.

2.1 Implant-based reconstruction

Implant-based breast reconstruction (IBR) represents a widely used surgical strategy for restoring breast contour after mastectomy. This method is favored for its relatively short operative time, avoidance of donor site morbidity, and compatibility with oncologic treatment schedules. IBR is particularly appropriate for patients with small-to-moderate breast volumes, preserved skin envelope integrity, and no significant systemic comorbidities. Key factors influencing the choice of technique include prior or anticipated radiotherapy, skin flap vascularity, patient preferences, and institutional protocols [16, 17, 27].

Typically, IBR is recommended for patients undergoing prophylactic mastectomies, such as BRCA mutation carriers, or those diagnosed with early-stage breast cancer who are not candidates for radiotherapy. It is also a practical option for patients who are not eligible for autologous reconstruction due to insufficient donor tissue, existing comorbidities that contraindicate lengthy procedures, or personal preference for less invasive alternatives [25].

Depending on the condition of the mastectomy flaps and planned oncologic treatments, IBR may be performed either at the time of the mastectomy (immediate) or postponed (delayed). Immediate reconstruction offers advantages in terms of emotional well-being and cosmetic outcome [20], while delayed reconstruction might be more appropriate when flap quality or adjuvant therapy pose risk for healing complications [18].

2.1.1 Two-stage (tissue expander and implant)

This method involves an initial procedure where a tissue expander (TE) is positioned either in the prepectoral or subpectoral plane and gradually inflated over weeks to accommodate the final implant volume. The progressive expansion of the skin and soft tissue envelope provides an opportunity to monitor flap viability and adjust surgical planning accordingly. Once sufficient expansion is achieved, a second operation is conducted to replace the expander with a permanent implant. The two-stage strategy remains a mainstay in implant-based reconstruction, particularly favored for patients at elevated risk of complications, such as those who require postmastectomy radiotherapy, have thinner skin flaps, or have comorbidities that may delay healing. By deferring the definitive implant placement, this approach offers time to assess the response to expansion and healing, reducing the likelihood of reconstructive failure [18, 20, 25].

Eligibility for this approach typically includes patients undergoing therapeutic mastectomy with questionable skin flap viability or those expected to receive adjuvant radiotherapy, where staging allows tissue remodeling and fibrosis stabilization. Additionally, patients with prior radiation exposure, elevated body mass index, smoking history, or diabetes may benefit from the gradual and adaptable nature of two-stage reconstruction, which facilitates more conservative decision-making and wound surveillance during expansion.

2.1.2 Direct-to-implant (DTI)

DTI technique consists of placing the definitive breast implant immediately after mastectomy, avoiding the need for a temporary tissue expander and the subsequent procedure. This method has gained popularity due to its ability to restore breast volume in a single stage, reduce the number of operative events, and enhance psychological recovery [23]. In appropriately selected cases, DTI reconstruction can shorten the overall surgical course and hospital stay, contributing to faster return to baseline activity [24].

Patients best suited for DTI are those undergoing prophylactic or therapeutic mastectomies who present with robust, well vascularized skin flaps and no current or anticipated need for postoperative radiotherapy. The quality and thickness of the mastectomy flaps are central to procedural success, as inadequate perfusion or flap atrophy significantly raises the risk of complications. Intraoperative assessment technologies, such as indocyanine green angiography, assist in real-time evaluation or perfusion to improve intraoperative decision making.

Additional favorable factors to DTI include the absence of significant comorbidities, such as uncontrolled diabetes or active smoking status, low to normal body mass index, and a surgical field unaltered by previous irradiation. DTI is particularly useful for patients preferring a less complex pathway, or when clinical and oncologic conditions support immediate reconstruction with delay. The ideal timing for DTI is synchronous with the mastectomy procedure, which facilitates immediate shaping of the reconstructed breast and potentially improves aesthetic results. Nevertheless, in patients where vascularity is questionable or systemic risk factors are present, a two-stage reconstruction may offer greater flexibility and safety margins [23, 24].

2.1.3 Prepectoral vs. subpectoral placement

Implant placement in breast reconstruction can follow two primary anatomical planes: beneath the pectoralis major muscle (subpectoral) or above it (prepectoral). The subpectoral technique has traditionally been the preferred approach due to the additional muscular coverage it offers, which may protect the implant and reduce the risk of exposure. However, it is not without defects. Patients often experience postoperative discomfort, muscle-related distortion of breast shape during contraction (animation deformity), and longer recovery periods [22].

In contrast, the prepectoral approach has gained favor in selected patients for its less invasive nature, reduced postoperative pain, and faster return to daily activities. Since it avoids disturbing the pectoral muscle, this technique eliminates the risk of animation deformity and offers improved esthetic outcomes, especially in cases of bilateral mastectomies or symmetrical reconstructions. However, successful outcomes depend heavily on the presence of thick, well-perfused mastectomy flaps. Thin or ischemic skin may increase the risk of complications such as flap necrosis and implant loss [22, 24, 26].

Patient selection for each plane of implant placement must be individualized. Subpectoral positioning may still favor patients with borderline vascularity, very thin flaps, or when additional soft tissue coverage is required for implant coverage. Conversely, prepectoral placement is optimal for patients with low risk complications, robust tissue perfusion, and sufficient flap thickness. Prepectoral reconstruction also demonstrates favorable outcomes in immediate reconstruction following nipple-sparing mastectomies, particularly when skin quality is preserved [24, 26].

For a timing perspective, both subpectoral and prepectoral approaches can be used in immediate or delayed settings. Nonetheless, the prepectoral technique is generally more appropriate when flap quality is excellent and postoperative radiotherapy is not anticipated. In irradiated or high-risk patients, the subpectoral approach or two-stage procedures are often preferred to reduce the incidence of complications and to allow for flap remodeling before definitive implant placement [22, 26].

2.1.4 Role of acellular dermal matrices (ADMs)

Acellular dermal matrices (ADMs) have become a cornerstone in modern IBR surgery due to their ability to reinforce the implant pocket and optimize contour outcomes. These biologically derived scaffolds offer mechanical support to the lower pole of the breast and contribute to improved implant stability, particularly in the prepectoral plane. ADMs facilitate implant coverage when soft tissue is insufficient and allow for more anatomic shaping of the reconstructed breast [19, 28].

Clinical data supports the use of ADMs in both immediate and two-stage reconstructions, where they have been associated with decreased rates of capsular contracture, improved symmetry, and enhanced esthetic results. Their application is particularly valuable in nipple-sparing mastectomies or when mastectomy flap thickness is borderline. Moreover, ADMs provide an additional layer of protection over the implant, especially in the prepectoral setting where muscle coverage is absent [28].

Several techniques exist for ADM placement, including complete anterior coverage of the implant, inferolateral hammock placement, or full wrapping. The choice of configuration depends on flap thickness, implant size, and surgeon experience. ADMs can also facilitate single-stage direct implant breast reconstruction (DTI) by compensating for the lack of muscle support, reducing the need for a second procedure in appropriately selected patients [28, 29].

However, the use of ADMs should be individualized based on the patient's clinical context. While advantageous, their use adds cost and may increase the risk of complications such as seroma, infection, or delayed wound healing, particularly in obese or diabetic patients. Careful patient selection, meticulous surgical technique, and adequate flap perfusion assessment are essential for optimizing outcomes.

2.1.5 Biological mesh

In addition to ADMs, there are materials such as bioabsorbable mesh composed of polydioxanone, designed to provide temporary reinforcement in revisionary breast surgery. Among these, Durasorb®, has been specifically evaluated in a prospective clinical series that demonstrated its ability to provide stable reinforcement during the healing phase. The mesh maintains mechanical strength for approximately 6 to 8 months before resorption, which aligns with the crucial period of tissue remodeling. The ideal candidates for Durasorb are patients undergoing revision procedures for implant malposition, capsular contracture, asymmetry, or recurrent ptosis. The mesh is typically placed during pocket repair, capsulorrhaphy, implant exchange, or mastopexy, where it functions as an internal scaffold to stabilize the reconstructed pocket. It is not recommended in cases of infection, uncontrolled seroma or severely compromised tissue quality, where biologic matrices may be more suitable. Clinical evidence supports these indications: in a prospective series of 17 patients and 27 breasts, Durasorb was used mainly to address malposition, contracture, asymmetry, and soft tissue laxity. After nearly 1 year of follow-up, no recurrences were observed, and complications were minimal-limited to a single seroma. No infections or healing problems occurred, and surgeons highlighted the ease of handling and fixation intraoperatively [30].

These results should be understood within the broader evolution of synthetic meshes in breast surgery. Early permanent material such as polypropylene or titanium-coated options offered support but were too rigid, often flattening the lower pole and altering breast contour. Braided absorbable meshes provided initial strength but carried higher infection risk, while rapidly resorbing options such a Vicryl® failed to give lasting reinforcement. Later, long-term absorbable monofilament meshes like poly-4-hidroxybutyrate (P4HB) advanced the field but were bulky for preprectoral applications [31].

Against this historical background, Durasorb represents the next-generation solution: fine, flexible, and specifically designed for breast surgery, combining durable support during the healing period with improved intraoperative handling and lower complication rates [30, 31].

2.1.6 Extracellular matrices derived from ovine tissue

Another alternative explored in implant-based breast reconstruction is the use of reinforced extracellular matrices derived from ovine tissue. Ovitex consists of multilayered ovine rumen stitched together with either absorbable or permanent polymer sutures, creating a biologic scaffold with added mechanical reinforcement. This design seeks to merge the remodeling capacity of biologic matrices with the structural durability typically associated with synthetics, while offering greater cost-effectiveness than human-derived ADMs.

In a single-surgeon longitudinal study that compared Ovitex with ADMs in two-stage, prepectoral expander-based reconstruction, no significant differences were observed in major or minor complications, implant loss, or overall reconstructive success. Outcomes were more closely linked to mastectomy flap viability than to mesh type. Importantly, Ovitex proved substantially more cost-effective (approximately 24–48% cheaper than human ADMs) while maintaining comparable safety and efficacy. The essential indications for Ovitex include patients undergoing immediate two-stage reconstruction after mastectomy, particularly when additional reinforcement of soft tissue is needed to support prepectoral tissue expanders. It is most appropriate in cases with adequate vascularized skin flaps, no prior radiation, and the absence of active infection or uncontrolled comorbidities. The mesh is typically placed at the time of the initial expander reconstruction, providing structural stability during the critical early healing phase (**Tables 1** and **2**) [32].

Material	Composition/structure	Essential indications	Surgical timing	Main outcomes	Cost/considerations
ADMs (e.g., Alloderm, Cortiva)	Human cadaveric acellular dermis	Pocket control, soft tissue reinforcement, reduction of capsular contracture; often used in prepectoral plane	At the time of immediate reconstruction (tissue expander or selected direct-to-implant)	Variable complications rates; reduction in contracture	High cost; significantly more expensive than ovine ECM.
Synthetic bioabsorbable mesh (Durasorb)	Synthetic monofilament bioabsorbable mesh (polydioxanone)	Revision cases: implant malposition, recurrent contracture, asymmetry, soft tissue ptosis (with adequate coverage, no infection)	During revision surgery: pocket repairs, capsulorrhaphy, implant exchange ± mastopexy	Very low complications (seroma)	Provides support for 6–8 months then resorbs; predictable, less costly than ADMs
Reinforced ovine ECM (Ovitex)	Multilayered ovine rumen reinforced with absorbable or permanent polymer sutures	Immediate two-stage prepectoral expander-based reconstruction in patients with well-vascularized flaps and no infection	At initial expander placement following mastectomy	Outcomes equivalent to ADMs; no significant differences in complications, implant loss, or reconstructive success	Cheaper than AlloDerm and Cortiva.

This table summarizes the main characteristics of acellular dermal matrices (ADMs), synthetic bioabsorbable mesh (Durasorb), and reinforced ovine extracellular matrix (Ovitex), highlighting their composition, and cost considerations. Adapted from Turin & Gutowski [30] and Sweitzer et al. [32].

Table 1.
Comparative features of ADMs, Durasorb, and Ovitex in implant-based breast reconstruction.

Parameters	Ovine ECM, n (%)	Human Cadaveric ADM, n (%)
Hematoma	9 (5.5)	1 (1.2)
Seroma	3 (1.8)	4 (4.9)
Infection	3 (1.8)	1 (1.2)
Mastectomy flap necrosis	4 (2.5)	6 (7.4)
Total	**19 (12.7)**	**12 (14.8)**
Implant loss	8 (4.9)	7 (8.6)
Implant replacement (initial RTOR)	11 (6.7	5 (6.2
Total	**19 (12.7)**	**12 (14.8)**
Total breasts	163	81

Reported surgical site complications in a patient population that received ovine ECM versus human cadaveric ADMs that required RTOR and recorded replacement or explant of implant. No differences were statistically significant. Implant replacement is an RTOR with washout and replacement of TE or implant at that time of washout secondary to hematoma or seroma.
Reproduced from Ref. [32]. Published under the Creative Commons Attribution–NonCommercial–NoDerivatives License (CC BY-NC-ND 4.0).

Table 2.
Major complications requiring return to the operating room (RTOR) in patients reconstructed with reinforced ovine ECM (Ovitex) versus human cadaveric ADMs.

2.2 Autologous reconstruction

Autologous breast reconstruction involves using the patient's own tissue, such as skin, fat, and muscle, to recreate a natural breast shape. It is considered the gold standard by many surgeons due to superior long-term esthetic outcomes, avoidance of implant-related complication and a more natural texture and aging process, albeit involving longer operative time and donor-site considerations [33].

2.2.1 TRAM: Pedicled and free (fTRAM)

TRAM flap, introduced in the early 1980s, may be harvested as a pedicled flap based on the superior epigastric vessels or as a free flap (fTRAM) using the deep inferior epigastric vessels. The pedicled version is technically simpler, demanding fewer microsurgical skills, but is associated with higher donor-site morbidity, including abdominal bulge and hernia formation [34]. In contrast, free TRAM flaps offer improved perfusion and greater flexibility in flap positioning, although both techniques sacrifice rectus muscle and may impair abdominal wall function.

Evidence from a prospective study of 42 patients (23 pedicled, 19 free TRAM) showed that although abdominal strength decreases transiently at 6 months, it generally recovers by 1 year; however, abdominal bulging was reported by 82% of free trial patients compared to 48% of those who had pedicled TRAMs [35]. A large retrospective comparison of pedicled TRAM *versus* DIEP flaps further demonstrated that DIEP reconstruction resulted in significantly lower rates of fat necrosis (17.7 vs. 58.5%), hernia (1.0 vs. 16.0%) and similar rates of abdominal bulge (9.4 vs. 14.9%) [36].

While pedicled TRAM flaps may yield slightly higher early breast satisfaction scores like BREAST-Q scale compared to free abdominal flaps, these differences tend to diminish after 3 years, with long-term satisfaction equalizing between groups [37].

Additionally, contemporary techniques such as muscle-sparing fTRAM and reinforcement of the donor site with onlay autografts have been effective in reducing morbidity without compromising esthetic outcomes [38].

2.2.2 DIEP and SIEA flaps

The DIEP flap, which spares the rectus abdominis muscle by selectively harvesting skin and fat based on the deep inferior epigastric perforators, significantly reduces donor-site complications such as hernia or abdominal weakness while maintaining core strength [39]. Meta-analyses and cohort data consistently show lower rates of fat necrosis, hernia, and bulging compared to muscle-sparing TRAM flaps, with a 20% lower risk of bulge [40].

A retrospective study from high-volume centers confirmed that DIEP flaps yield high reliability, with flap survival rates exceeding 98%, and fewer donor-site morbidities in experienced centers [41]. Recent data also emphasize that using medial row perforators reduces postoperative abdominal bulging, particularly in patients with preoperative rectus diastasis (>2 cm) [42]. This flap has become widely adopted as the preferred technique in many high-volume microsurgery centers due to excellent outcomes and patient satisfaction.

The SIEA flap avoids dissection of the rectus sheath altogether, offering the lowest donor-site morbidity. However, its anatomical variability limits its use; in one multicenter cohort of 720 patients, the SIEA group had significantly higher rates of donor-site complications (over 50%) compared to DIEP (about 28%), including seroma, wound dehiscence, and infection, despite slightly better abdominal physical well-being scores at 1 year [43]. Moreover, a cohort study of 169 free flaps (44 SIEA vs. 125 DIEP) reported higher rates of arterial insufficiency (14 vs. 1%), re-exploration, and complete flap failure (14 vs. 2%) in the SIEA group [44].

A recent institution-level analysis of 628 abdominal flaps (2017–2023) of 571 DIEP and 67 SIEA found similar overall donor-site outcomes between DIEP and SIEA, but a statistically higher rate of arterial thrombosis in superficial-system flaps (4.5 vs. 0.7%, $p = 0.015$), underscoring increased vascular risk with SIEA despite comparable failure rates [45].

2.2.3 Latissimus dorsi and thoracodorsal artery perforator (TDAP) flap

The Latissimus Dorsi (LD) flap, traditionally used as a pedicled musculocutaneous flap, remains a reliable option for breast reconstruction, particularly in patients with insufficient abdominal tissue, prior abdominoplasty, or post-radiation needs. A large 18-year-single-surgeon cohort of 142 LD reconstructions reported seroma as the most frequent donor-site complication at 26%, yet flap loss was very rare and patient satisfaction remained high [46].

A novel variation, the dorsoepigastric flap (a muscle-sparing LD-based flap), was anatomically characterized by Jimenez Muñoz Ledo and Haddad Tame and preserves most of the muscle as well as allow to carry a wide cutaneous island, who reported minimal donor site morbidity and complication in an initial pilot cohort, suggesting this approach as a promising alternative in selected cases [47].

Despite these strengths, LD flap harvesting can impair shoulder function, with reductions in strength (up to 21% in extension and adduction) documented up to 12 months postoperatively. However, daily activities typically remain unaffected, and the use of split-LD or nerve-sparing techniques can mitigate functional deficits [48].

The thoracodorsal artery perforator (TDAP) flap which harvests skin and fat over the back, without sacrificing muscle, offers robust flap viability up to 98%, minimal donor-site morbidity and reliable use in both irradiated and non-irradiated reconstructions, with complication rates around 19% in large series [49]. **Figure 1** more recent surgical refinements for the TDAP flap include delayed elevation to enhance vessel caliber, as well as propeller-style flap design and applications for the total breast reconstruction in patients lacking abdominal donor tissue (**Figure 1**) [50].

2.2.4 Profunda artery perforator (PAP) flap

The profunda artery perforator (PAP) flap has become an increasingly reliable option for autologous breast reconstruction, especially in patients for whom abdominal donor sites are unavailable or non-viable. It provides well-vascularized tissue with low donor-site morbidity, concealed scars along the posterior thigh crease, and high esthetic satisfaction rates [51, 52]. Clinical series have consistently reported excellent flap survival and outcomes, establishing that PAP flap as a dependable secondary choice when DIEP is contraindicated [53].

Anatomical refinements have improved preoperative planning. Largo et al. proposed a systematic mapping strategy of PAP perforators, facilitating reproducible flap design with no flap loss in their clinical cohort [54]. Moreover, novel designs such as the diagonal PAP (dPAP) have been shown to increase harvested tissue volume without elevating complication rates [55].

PAP flap offers several advantages, including providing well-vascularized tissue with reliable pedicle length and caliber, and minimal donor-site morbidity. Furthermore, it can be harvested bilaterally or in combination with other flaps when larger volume is required [51, 56]. Nevertheless, limitations exist. The volume is generally smaller than that achievable with abdominal-based flaps such as DIEP, which may restrict its use in patients requiring larger reconstructions. In addition, donor-site complications, such as wound dehiscence, seroma, or contour irregularities, can occur, although their incidence remains relatively low [52, 53].

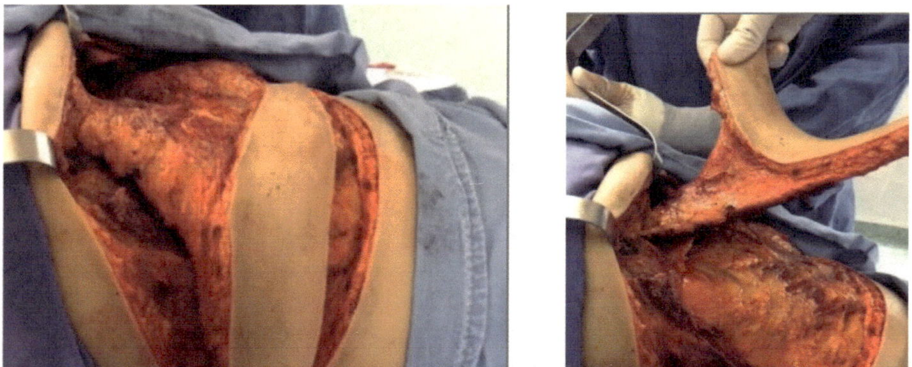

Figure 1.
Design of the dorsoepigastric flap. Reproduced with permission from Ref. [47].

2.2.5 Transverse upper gracilis (TUG) flap

The transverse upper gracilis flap is a myocutaneous flap harvested from the medial thigh, incorporating the gracilis muscle and its overlying skin paddle. It is based on perforators from the ascending branch of the medial circumflex femoral artery, providing a reliable vascular supply with a pedicle length of approximately 6–8 cm. The flap is designed transversely along the upper inner thigh crease, which allows for primary closure and well-concealed donor-site scars. Its harvest is usually performed with the patient in the supine frog-leg position, which can facilitate simultaneous breast reconstruction [57, 58].

The TUG flap offers several advantages: it provides well-vascularized tissue with consistent anatomy, and the gracilis muscle harvest contributes additional bulk in the early postoperative period. Donor-site morbidity is generally low, and the resulting scar can mimic a cosmetic thigh-lift incision.

However, the limitations include reduced available tissue volume compared with abdominal flaps, which restricts its use in larger reconstructions. Additionally flap atrophy over time may occur due to the resorption of gracilis muscle, potentially compromising long-term volume retention. Other challenges include the shorted pedicle length [59, 60].

2.2.6 Inferior gluteal artery perforator (IGAP) and superior gluteal artery perforator (SGAP) flaps

The advent of perforator flaps has transformed breast reconstruction by allowing the transfer of autologous tissue with minimal donor site morbidity. When the abdomen is not viable for a DIEP flap, either due to previous surgeries, limited tissue availability, or patient preference, gluteal flaps are a reliable alternative. Among them, the IGAP and SGAP stand out, both described in the 1990s by Allen et al., as an evolution of gluteal myocutaneous flaps [61].

IGAP flap is based on inferior gluteal artery perforators, with a 7–10 cm long pedicle. The skin is designed along the gluteal fold, which allows for scar concealment and improved contour in patients with saddlebag deformity. Its oblique course through the gluteus maximus increases the complexity of the dissection. The scar can be hidden under underwear or a swimsuit, although the donor site may present a flattening of the upper gluteus [62]. Both flaps preserve gluteus maximus function, reduce the risk of sciatic nerve injury compared to traditional myocutaneous flaps, and require high microsurgical expertise.

In the accumulated clinical experience with IGAP and SGAP flaps, the risk of the nerve injury is low; however, IGAP flaps may be associated with greater pain when sitting and a higher risk of dehiscence in bilateral reconstructions, whereas SGAP flaps can result in flattening of the upper buttock [62]. The overall safety profile of the IGAP flap has been further evaluated in a recent proportional meta-analysis of 239 IGAP flaps, which reported a total flap loss rate of 3%, partial flap loss of 2%, a hematoma rate of 3%, donor-site complications in 15% of cases, and an overall complication rate of 40%, supporting its reliability as an option for autologous breast reconstruction [63].

Indications for the use of gluteal artery perforator flaps include patients without available abdominal donor tissue, those with excess gluteal adiposity, non-smokers, and individuals without prior liposuction in the donor area [62]. The advantages of these flaps are the provision of adequate adipose volume, well-concealed scars, and preservation of muscle function. Nevertheless, there are important limitations, such as the

Characteristic	SGAP (Superior gluteal artery perforator)	IGAP (Inferior gluteal artery perforator)
Pedicle length	5–8 cm [62]	7–10 cm (longer) [62]
Flap location	Upper buttock region	Gluteal fold (crease)
Scar position	Can be concealed under underwear or swimwear [62]	Hidden within the gluteal crease [62]
Tissue volume	Moderate	Moderate to high, useful in patients with "saddlebag deformity" [62]
Donor-site contour	Risk of flattening of the upper buttock [62]	Improved contour of lateral thigh and lower buttock [62]
Postoperative comfort	Less pain when sitting	More discomfort and higher risk of dehiscence in bilateral reconstructions [62]
Nerve morbidity	Low risk of nerve injury	Low risk; occasional division of small sensory nerves [62]
Ideal candidates	Patients with excess tissue in the upper buttock, unsuitable for abdominal flaps	Patients with large buttocks, preference for scar hidden in gluteal fold [62]

This table summarizes the main comparative characteristics of the superior gluteal artery perforator (SGAP) and inferior gluteal artery perforator (IGAP) flaps in autologous breast reconstruction. Adapted from Ref. [62].

Table 3.
Comparative characteristics of SGAP and IGAP flaps.

technical complexity of the procedure, less favorable positioning for bilateral reconstructions, and sitting discomfort particularly associated with IGAP flaps (**Table 3**).

2.2.7 Lateral thigh perforator (LTP) flap

The lateral thigh perforator (LTP) flap is based on septocutaneous perforators arising from the ascending branch of the lateral circumflex femoral artery, located in the posterior septum between the tensor fasciae latae (TFL) and gluteus medius. It evolved from the tensor fasciae latae myocutaneous flap into a pure perforator flap, and has gained recognition as an alternative when the abdomen is not suitable (e.g., minimal adipose tissue, previous abdominal surgery, or patient preference). In 2012, the septocutaneous variant was described, and the term "LTP" was later adopted to improve patient comprehension [64].

Anatomy, planning, and indications

- Perforators: Septocutaneous, located in the posterior septum between TFL and gluteus medius.
- Pedicle length: typically 6–8 cm, with vessel calibers compatible with the internal mammary system.
- Preoperative planning: MRA is routinely performed to identify perforators; intraoperative Doppler confirms their location.
- Positioning: Supine throughout the procedure, allowing simultaneous harvest and recipient-site preparation by two or three surgical teams.
- Ideal candidates: Women unsuitable for abdominal flaps, those with lateral thigh lipodystrophy, or those who prefer to avoid abdominal scar [64].

Dissection is performed suprafascially over the TFL, with careful identification of the lateral femoral cutaneous nerve along the anterior border. The fascia is incised longitudinally at the posterior septum, and dissection proceeds toward the ascending branch of the LCFA. Anastomosis is performed end- to-end to internal mammary vessels, with venous couplers commonly used (2.0 mm). Donor-site closure involves triple-layer quilting sutures to minimize seroma and dehiscence; flap width is limited [64].

The LTP flap is a reliable, versatile, and reproducible option for autologous breast reconstruction when abdominal flaps are unavailable. Large prospective series report very low total flap loss (~1–2%), minimal recipient site morbidity, and dramatic reductions in donor-site complications with straightforward refinements [64, 65].

2.2.8 Lumbar artery perforator (LAP) flap

The LAP flap is a fasciocutaneous free flap based on profunda lumbar perforators (typically L2-L4) that arise from the dorsal branches of the lumbar arteries and course through or between the erector spinae and quadratus lumborum to supply the posterior flank and lower back integument. Preoperative CTA reliably maps one or two dominant perforators-commonly at the L4 level-and defines intramuscular course and caliber, which average 1–2 mm at the perforator and 2–3 mm at the pedicle, with pedicle lengths often 6–8 cm. Patient positioning is usually prone or lateral for harvest with supine microvascular inset; some centers perform simultaneous bilateral harvests with staged or immediate inset using a defined sequence to limit ischemia. Dissection proceeds in the subfascial plane, skeletonizing the perforator to the source vessel; neurotization using the superior cluneal nerve to an anterior intercostal branch is optional for sensate reconstruction. Anastomosis is typical of the internal mammary system (often with composite DIEA/DIEV grafts or pedicle extensions when additional length is required), and stacked or conjoined LAPs can be employed for unilateral volume [66].

Contemporary series report high reliability. In a 108-flap consecutive experience of simultaneous bilateral LAPS, overall flap success was ~97%, with significant complications ~23%; intraoperative hypotension/hypothermia correlated with arterial thrombosis or postoperative compromise. Early institutional series of simultaneous bilateral cases reported 1 total loss among 60 flaps, with mean ischemia ~90 min and routine use of composite vein/artery grafts. Donor-site issues include seroma, delayed wound healing at the posterior waistline, contour asymmetry, and neuropathic discomfort along cluneal distributions; abdominal wall morbidity is avoided. Recipient-site complications mirror other perforator flaps (take-back for congestion or thrombosis, fat necrosis, with rates comparable to PAP/MG in most reports) [67].

Ideal candidates are patients without adequate abdominal tissue (prior abdominoplasty, thin habitus) who carry substantial flank/lumbar adiposity that yields favorable breast shape and projection. Advantages include hidden posterior-oblique scar and muscle preservation; limitations are a short/variable pedicle, challenging exposure in the lower back, and logistics of position changes in bilateral cases. Routine CTA is recommended to select the dominant perforator(s) and plan incision length to allow primary closure (often ≤10 cm width, larger in lax patients). Strategies to mitigate risk include meticulous thermal management, hemodynamic stability, liberal use of pedicle extension/composite grafts when needed, and consideration of staged bilateral reconstruction in select patients or centers early in the learning curve.

Compared with PAP, LAP often provides thicker, more projection-friendly tissue; compared with SGAP/IGAP, donor morbidity is generally lower but pedicle length is shorter [68].

As summarized in **Table 4**, the main autologous breast reconstruction flaps are compared. This overview highlights the versatility of non-abdominal donor sites while also underscoring the specific technical challenges and anatomical considerations.

2.3 Hybrid techniques

Hybrid techniques in breast reconstruction combine the advantages of both implant-based and autologous approaches to optimize esthetic outcomes, particularly in patients with limited donor tissue or prior radiation. These strategies may involve the use of fat grafting to refine contour and enhance soft-tissue coverage, or the combination of flaps with implants to achieve volume and symmetry. Hybrid reconstruction has gained increasing popularity due to its versatility, ability to reduce implant-related complications, and potential to improve patient satisfaction in complex reconstructive scenarios.

2.3.1 Fat grafting/lipofilling

Autologous fat grafting (AFG), or lipofilling, has emerged as a versatile tool for volume restoration and contour refinement following breast reconstruction. A 2025 study of 12,078 patients across 12 studies found that cell-assisted lipotransfer (CAL) and Platelet rich plasm (PRP) assisted techniques significantly improve fat graft survival rates compared to conventional fat grafting, without increasing complication risk [70]. Additionally, studies show no increase in locoregional recurrence when fat grafting was used within 2 years-post mastectomy, except among those with lymph node involvement [71]. Fat grafting is also effective in alleviating post-mastectomy pain syndrome (PMPS). Key advantages include a natural contour, high patient acceptance,

Flaps	**DIEP**	**SGAP**	**IGAP**	**LTP**	**PAP**	**TUG**	**LAP**
Dissection difficulty	Low	High	Moderate	Low	Moderate	Low	High
Pedicle caliber mismatch	No	Yes	Yes	No	Yes	Yes	Yes
Need for position changes	No	Yes	Yes	No	No	No	Yes
Sensitivity	Lower intercostal nerves	Superior cluneal nerves	Branches of inferior gluteal nerve (S1–S2)	Lateral femoral cutaneous nerve	Posterior femoral cutaneous nerve	Cutaneous branches of the obturator nerve	Superior cluneal nerves

DIEP, deep inferior epigastric perforator; SGAP, superior gluteal artery perforator; IGAP, inferior gluteal artery perforator; LTP, lateral thigh perforator; PAR profunda artery perforator; TUG, transverse upper gracilis; LAP, lumbar artery perforator.
Reproduced from Ref. [69], under the Creative Commons Attribution-NonCommercial-NoDerivs 4.0 International License (CC BY-NC-ND 4.0).

Table 4.
Characteristics of autologous breast reconstruction flaps.

and minimal invasiveness, which are oncologically safe in most reconstructive settings and can improve contour irregularities and implant coverage. Reported disadvantages include variable graft retention rates, as well as the risk of oil cysts, calcification, infection and fat necrosis and need for multiple sessions in some cases [72].

2.3.2 Combination of implant and autologous tissue

Hybrid breast reconstruction combining implants with autologous fat grafting has gained prominence for patients requiring greater volume or improved contour in cases where flaps alone are insufficient. A 2022 systematic review showed that hybrid approaches improve esthetic outcomes, reduce contour deformities and lower reconstructive failure rates compared to implant-only reconstruction, especially in irradiated patients [73].

In this context, the concept of lipoframing, developed by Jimenez Muñoz-Ledo et al., offers a comprehensive approach that integrates preaxillary, lateral, and inframammary liposuction with precise fat grafting to enhance better shape. In a retrospective cohort of 554 patients, including both esthetic and reconstructive cases, satisfaction rates were (92%), with improved breast symmetry in 89% of patients and low complication rate 5%. This technique is particularly valuable in postmastectomy reconstruction, where it improves natural breast contour, reducing implant visibility or rippling [74, 75].

3. Surgical timing considerations

3.1 Immediate vs. delayed reconstruction

In the context of postmastectomy radiation therapy (PMRT), the timing of autologous breast reconstruction plays a pivotal role in optimizing outcomes and minimizing complications. Although immediate reconstruction offers psychological and esthetic advantages, exposure of a newly reconstructed breast to radiation has been associated with higher rates of fat necrosis, fibrosis, and need for revisions. As a result, delayed reconstruction has become a widely accepted approach for patients who require PMRT.

The study by Arnautovic et al., evaluated outcomes of 303 patients undergoing delayed microvascular breast reconstruction at different time intervals after PMRT. The analysis revealed no statistically significant difference in major complications rates among patients who underwent reconstruction within 12 months, between 12 and 18 months, or beyond. The risk of complications appeared when peak reconstruction was performed within the first 6 months post PMRT [25].

Based on these findings, the authors suggest that delayed microvascular reconstruction can be safely initiated as early as 6 months after the completion of PMRT, provided careful patient selection. Immediate reconstruction remains a viable option in select patients not undergoing PMRT. The timing decision should be individualized, integrating oncologic plans, patient comorbidities, tissue quality, and psychosocial preferences to optimize surgical esthetic outcomes [25].

3.2 Impact of postmastectomy radiation therapy (PMRT)

Postmastectomy radiation therapy (PMRT) is a critical component of breast cancer treatment, reducing locoregional recurrence and improving survival in high risk patients; however, its impact on breast reconstruction, particularly autologous reconstruction, is significant. Radiation can impair wound healing, cause fibrosis and affect the vascularity and pliability of the skin and underlying tissue. These complications have led many surgeons to delay autologous reconstruction until after the completion of PMRT. However modern radiation techniques with three dimensional planning have improved targeting and minimized damage to surrounding tissues. Wu Young et al. compared outcomes between immediate and delayed autologous breast reconstruction in patients receiving PMRT and evaluated wound dehiscence. This suggests that immediate reconstruction may be feasible and safe in select patients undergoing PMRT, challenging prior assumptions [76].

3.3 Optimal timing after PMRT: Evidence from recent studies

Timing of delayed reconstruction following PMRT remains controversial, with prior beliefs favoring prolonged delay to minimize complications. Arnautovic evaluated and the study found no statistically significant difference in major complication rates across these time frames, including fat necrosis, fat loss, or wound healing issues [25].

However a slight peak in complication rates was observed between 2 and 6 months post PMRT, suggesting a potential window of vulnerability. Based on these findings, the authors support proceeding with reconstruction as early as 6 months after PMRT, with close patient monitoring and individualized risk assessment. This flexibility enables faster recovery and improved quality of life while maintaining flap safety [76].

3.4 Implications for microvascular flap success

The studies reported no cases of total flap loss in either immediate or delayed groups and found comparable rates of fat necrosis and surgical site infections. Importantly, the immediate reconstruction group required fewer revision surgeries, suggesting more stable outcomes when performed concurrently with mastectomy [76].

However, Parmeshwar et al., showed that timing of PMRT did not significantly impact free flap outcomes or need for revision surgeries. Those with PMRT of tissue expander prior autologous reconstruction experienced significantly more complications overall and average. For 34.7% of patients who planned for autologous flap reconstruction from initial consultation, radiation after the flap may have improved their overall outcomes. As added complications cause delays in cancer therapy and final reconstruction, the result of the flap when possible may improve the overall experience for breast cancer patients [77].

4. Factors affecting the outcome

Postoperative complications following breast reconstruction represent a critical determinant of both esthetic outcome and patient satisfaction. Understanding the most frequent complications, their risk factors, and predictive tools is essential for surgical planning and patient counseling.

The common postoperative complications are described here:

1. *Seroma*: Occurs in up to 20% of implant-based reconstructions and is especially frequent with acellular dermal matrix (ADM) use. Seromas may delay adjuvant

DOI: http://dx.doi.org/10.5772/intechopen.1013807

therapy, lead to infection, or result in implant loss. Key risk factors include high BMI (>30 kg/m^2), ADM usage, and prior radiotherapy. Preventive strategies include quilting sutures, elimination of dead space, early drain removal, and tissue expander designs with integrated drainage ports. Treatment typically involves ultrasound-guided aspiration or drainage; refractory or infected cases may require surgical intervention [78, 79].

2. *Hematoma:* Incidence approximates 2–10%, primarily within the first 24–72 hours postoperatively. Presents with swelling, pain, and discoloration. Large hematomas increase risk of infection, fat necrosis, and capsular contracture. Prompt surgical evacuation mitigates complications.

3. *Surgical site infection:* Ranges from superficial cellulitis to deep infections that may necessitate implant removal. Risk increases in patients with diabetes, smoking history, radiotherapy exposure, and hematoma. Infections are a leading cause of reconstructive failure.

4. *Wound dehiscence:* Partial or full separation of incision edges, often due to tension, ischemia, infection, or poor healing. Minor cases may heal by secondary intention, whereas major dehiscence may require surgical closure and carries risk of implant or flap exposure.

5. *Skin flap necrosis:* Affects 4–14% of patients after mastectomy with immediate reconstruction; up to 41% in some series depending on definition and detection of minor necrosis. It occurs due to inadequate perfusion of mastectomy skin flaps. Risk factors include smoking, obesity, diabetes, nipple-sparing technique, and preoperative radiotherapy. Indocyanine green (ICG) angiography can predict areas of hypoperfusion and reduce necrosis rates. Management ranges from local wound care to debridement or flap revision.

6. *Capsular contracture:* Occurs following implant-based reconstruction and represents fibrotic encapsulation leading to firmness, distortion, and discomfort. Incidence estimated at 10–16%, though reduced (2–4%) when meshes or biologic matrices are used. Associated risk factors include hematoma, infection, implant surface, and subglandular placement. Severe cases often require capsulectomy and implant exchange.

7. *Implant loss/flap failure:* Implant-based failures are most commonly due to infection, exposure, or necrosis; autologous flap failures partial or total occur in under 5% of cases, usually due to vascular thrombosis. Early detection and prompt surgical intervention may enable salvage.

8. *Fat necrosis:* Frequently develops in autologous reconstructions, particularly in large-volume flaps or irradiated fields. Clinically presented as firm nodules that can mimic recurrence. Diagnosis by imaging or biopsy; most cases are benign and resolve spontaneously (**Table 5**).

9. *Delayed wound healing:* Common in patients with obesity, diabetes, malnutrition, or prior radiation. Manifests as prolonged drainage, slow epithelialization, or tissue breakdown. Often necessitates advanced wound care or surgical revision.

Complication	Incidence	Key risk factors	Typical management
Seroma	~5–20%	BMI > 30, ADM use, radiotherapy	Drainage / aspiration, quilting sutures
Hematoma	~2–10%	Poor hemostasis, surgical factors	Prompt evacuation
Infection	~5–25%	Diabetes, smoking, prior radiation, hematoma	Antibiotics ± explantation
Wound dehiscence	~3–20%	Flap necrosis, tension, infection	Local care or reclosure
Skin flap necrosis	~4–14% (up to 41%)	Smoking, obesity, diabetes, NSM, radiation	Debridement, flap revision
Capsular contracture	~10–16% (mesh 2–4%)	Hematoma, infection, implant plane	Capsulectomy, implant exchange
Implant loss / flap failure	<5% (flaps)	Infection, necrosis, vascular complications	Explantation or surgical salvage
Fat necrosis	~10–40%	Large flaps, irradiation	Imaging follow-up, biopsy if indicated
Delayed healing	Variable	Obesity, diabetes, poor nutrition, radiation	Advanced wound care, possible reoperation

Table 5.
Complications and associated risk factors compiled from high-impact studies and recent systematic reviews in plastic and reconstructive surgery literature.

4.1 Impact of comorbidities (diabetes, hypertension, obesity)

Recent literature strongly supports the role of comorbidities particularly obesity, diabetes, and hypertension as significant predictors of postoperative complications in breast reconstruction procedures [80, 81].

- Obesity (BMI >30 kg/m^2) is independently associated with:
- Increased surgical complications (Odds Ratio [OR] 2.29)
- Higher rate of medical complications (OR 2.89)
- Greater need for reoperation (OR 1.91)
- Wound dehiscence (OR 2.51)

A 2022 meta-analysis found that obesity, hypertension, diabetes, and smoking had cumulative effects on complications in breast reconstruction. Particularly in metabolically unhealthy obesity, these comorbidities significantly increased wound and flap-related complications, especially when operative time exceeded 4 hours [82, 83]. Despite increased risks, some studies suggest that morbidly obese patients can safely undergo prepectoral breast reconstruction with acceptable complication rates [84, 85]:

- Skin necrosis: 3.5%,
- Wound dehiscence: 5.9%,

- Seroma: 4.7%,
- Reconstruction failure: 1.2%.

4.2 Role of preoperative optimization

Breast reconstruction surgery is a complex procedure whose success depends not only on the surgical technique used but also on the patient's systemic conditions. Therefore, it is essential to carry out a thorough preoperative assessment to identify and address clinical risk factors that could negatively impact wound healing, compromise tissue integrity, or even lead to reconstructive failure (**Table 6**) [81].

4.2.1 Comprehensive evaluation and risk stratification

The general health status and comorbidities should be assessed through a thorough medical history. Conditions such as diabetes, hypertension, and obesity must be well controlled. Obesity is a known risk factor for complications (level of evidence 1). Smoking increases the risk of complications and should therefore be discouraged. Some factors cannot be modified, such as prior or planned radiotherapy, as well as the type and stage of cancer. The physical examination should evaluate the availability of tissue in donor areas such as the back, abdomen, thighs, and buttocks, as well as the condition of the recipient site, including skin quality [83].

4.2.2 Diabetes mellitus: Risk profile and implications in breast reconstruction

Diabetes mellitus (DM) represents a significant systemic comorbidity that has been strongly correlated with an increased likelihood of postoperative complications in breast reconstruction procedures. Among these, wound dehiscence appears as the most consistently reported adverse outcome. Although the presence of diabetes does not appear to markedly elevate the risk of total flaps loss or surgical site infection, there is robust evidence linking it to higher rates of wound breakdown.

A recent meta-analysis by Mortada et al., which evaluated data from more than 19,000 patients undergoing breast reconstruction, demonstrated a statistically significant increase in wound dehiscence among diabetic individuals, regardless of whether their blood glucose levels were reasonably controlled [81]. This suggests that even mild or well-managed diabetes may impair tissue healing and surgical outcomes.

Condition	Preoperative recommendation
Diabetes mellitus	Maintain HbA1c below 7%; ensure endocrinology consultation and intensive perioperative monitoring [81]
Obesity	Aim for BMI <30; initiate supervised weight loss programs and implement thromboembolic prophylaxis [86]
Smoking	Complete cessation ≥4 weeks pre- and postoperatively; include behavioral and pharmacologic support [79]
Hypertension	Optimize blood pressure control, ideally <140/90 mmHg before surgery [83]
Prior radiotherapy	Plan delayed autologous reconstruction when possible; avoid prepectoral implant placement unless skin is thick and well vascularized [22]

Table 6.
Preoperative optimization recommendations for breast reconstruction candidates.

The underlying pathophysiology is multifactorial and includes tissue hypoxia, microvascular dysfunction, and chronic low-grade inflammation, all of which contribute to delayed wound healing and an increased susceptibility to mechanical failure of the incision. Hyperglycemia also disrupts collagen synthesis and compromises leukocyte function, further compounding the risk of postoperative complications.

Current recommendations for reconstructive surgery suggest achieving a target Hba1c level below 7%, accompanied by strict glycemic monitoring during the perioperative period. This preoperative optimization becomes especially critical for reconstructions, where even minor metabolic dysfunctions may result in partial or total flap loss [81, 83].

4.2.3 Obesity: Risk and surgical considerations in reconstructive planning

Obesity is widely recognized as a significant risk factor for postoperative complications in breast reconstruction. Individuals with a body mass index (BMI) of 30 or higher demonstrate an elevated likelihood of developing adverse outcomes such as surgical site infections, seromas, hematomas, and reconstructive failure [86].

Beyond systemic complications, obesity has also been linked to a higher incidence of donor-site morbidity. While the DIEP flap is generally preferred due to its muscle-sparing nature, evidence from Egeberg et al. indicates that even this technique may not fully mitigate the risk of abdominal bulging or hernia in obese patients [40]. Moreover, previous research by Chang et al. underscores that obesity itself is an independent predictor of abdominal wall complications, regardless of the flap type selected [85].

4.2.4 Smoking: Vasoconstriction and risk of tissue necrosis

Tobacco use adversely affects wound healing and tissue viability through mechanisms that involve persistent vasoconstriction, impaired angiogenesis, and heightened proinflammatory activity. These pathophysiological alterations result in a significant reduction in tissue perfusion, increasing the likelihood of partial flap necrosis and wound breakdown. Clinical evidence from large-scale, multicenter cohort studies has demonstrated that active smoking is strongly associated with elevated postoperative complication rates in plastic and reconstructive surgery, including infection, delayed wound healing, and increased need for surgical revision [25, 79, 87].

Due to these risks, complete smoking cessations is strongly advised for at least 4 weeks before and after surgery. Behavioral counseling and, when appropriate, pharmacologic interventions should be implemented to support abstinence and improve surgical outcomes. Furthermore, clinical practice guidelines consider smoking a relative contraindication for immediate breast reconstruction, given its negative impact on both implant- and flap-based techniques [65].

4.2.5 Radiation therapy: Planning of timing and technique

Postmastectomy radiation therapy (PMRT) induces a series of detrimental histological changes in the chest wall, including dermal fibrosis, microvascular atrophy, and decreased tissue compliance. These alterations significantly impair the outcomes of breast reconstruction, particularly when implants are used. In irradiated patients who undergo implant-based reconstruction, systematic reviews have shown

DOI: http://dx.doi.org/10.5772/intechopen.1013807

a markedly increased risk of complications such as infections, capsular contracture, and implant loss [22].

Due to these well-documented risks, immediate reconstruction in patients with planned PRMT is generally discouraged. Instead, delayed reconstruction using autologous tissue is recommended, with flaps such as DIEP or latissimus dorsi offering superior long-term outcomes and greater resistance to radiation-induced fibrosis [20, 27]. These techniques have demonstrated lower complication rates and higher patient satisfaction compared to implant-based approaches in the context of prior radiation [27].

In patients who have already received radiation therapy, prepectoral implant placement should be avoided unless the skin flap is adequately thick (≥1 cm) and demonstrates robust vascularity, as thin irradiated skin significantly increases the risk of flap necrosis and implant exposure [22].

Emerging data suggest that delayed microvascular reconstruction can be performed safely as early as 6 months after PMRT, with no significant increase in flap loss or systemic complications, provided proper patient selection and institutional experience [25].

Thus, the timing and method of reconstruction in irradiated patients must be highly individualized, taking into account the radiation field, skin quality, reconstructive goals, and institutional resources.

4.3 Readmission rates and surgical site infection risks

Readmission rates are an important factor to take into consideration. Readmission in the first 30 days postoperation is a common indicator of complications. Readmission rates range from 4 to 12%, and these numbers can increase with more complex procedures, comorbidities like diabetes, hypertension, and obesity.

Hospital readmission remains a critical quality and safety metric in reconstructive breast surgery. A study using the Nationwide Readmissions Database (NRD) involving 15,325 cases reported a 90-day readmission rate of 8.7%, with 8.4% for autologous and 9.06% for implant-based reconstructions, where infection was the leading cause of readmission [79]. Another large study using ACS-NSQIP data of 3097 patients showed a 30-day readmission rate of 5.8%, with significant predictors, including obesity (OR 1.62), smoking (OR 1.60), and longer operative times [87, 88].

Surgical site infections are also a topic to consider in this type of surgery. This complication ranges from a 2 to 10% of total cases, and it usually depends on the reconstructive method used. Also depends on the patients' risk factor; like comorbidities diabetes and hypertension, personal hygiene, smoking and others.

5. Outcome measures and patient satisfaction

5.1 Esthetic and psychosocial benefits

Post-mastectomy breast reconstruction is not only a physical intervention but a complex process of emotional and identity restoration. Current literature confirms that esthetic outcomes are intrinsically linked to psychosocial dimensions, significantly impacting body image, self-esteem, sexuality, and perception of normalcy.

Qualitative studies have shown that patients frequently report a sense of being "whole again" after reconstruction, which translates into better emotional adjustment and reintegration into social life [89]. Comparative studies between mastectomy-only patients and those who underwent immediate or delayed reconstruction report higher scores in body image, self-worth, and sexual function among the reconstructed groups [90, 91].

A recent systematic review suggests that immediate reconstruction may offer superior short-term psychosocial benefits, although these differences tend to equalize in the long term, suggesting that the timing of quality-of-life assessment may influence perceived outcomes [91].

5.2 BREAST-Q and other validated tools

The BREAST-Q has emerged as the most validated and specific tool for evaluating outcomes in post-mastectomy patients. It measures domains such as psychosocial, sexual, and physical well-being, as well as satisfaction with the breast and medical care. Its modular design allows application at various stages of treatment, from preoperative evaluation to long-term follow-up.

Compared to general instruments such as the SF-36, EORTC QLQ-BR23, or FACT-B, the BREAST-Q offers more sensitive and clinically meaningful data, particularly in plastic surgery. It addresses critical aspects such as perceived naturalness, symmetry, and restoration of body image [92]. Its response to clinically significant changes has been validated in multicenter studies, and its widespread use has helped tailor care protocols around patient satisfaction.

5.3 Long-term results: Autologous vs. implant-based methods

The long-term outcomes of breast reconstruction can be broadly categorized into two primary approaches: autologous reconstruction, using the patient's own tissue, and implant-based reconstruction, typically with silicone or saline prosthesis. Both methods offer unique advantages and trade-offs that influence long-term satisfaction, complications rates, and quality of life.

Several studies have shown that autologous reconstruction is associated with higher long-term satisfaction, particularly in domains such as breast softness, natural appearance, and body image [92, 93]. Patients who undergo flap-based reconstruction (e.g., DIEP or TRAM flaps) consistently report more stable outcomes over time and fewer concerns with implant-related complications such as capsular contracture, rupture, or need for replacement surgeries [94].

In contrast, implant-based reconstruction often involves shorter initial surgery times, avoids donor site morbidity, and is more widely accessible. However, satisfaction with implant-based reconstruction tends to decline over time, particularly when patients experience complications or feel dissatisfaction with esthetic symmetry or tactile quality [4, 93]. Moreover, some studies have highlighted increased anxiety related to implant integrity and long-term surveillance.

A systematic review by Tsantakis et al. indicates that although both methods improve quality of life and psychosocial outcomes compared to mastectomy alone, autologous reconstruction tends to provide more sustained improvements, especially beyond the two-yes postoperative period [91]. The BREAST-Q score in this cohort favored autologous methods in domains such as sexual well-being, psychosocial adjustment, and satisfaction with breasts.

From an oncologic safety standpoint, no significant difference in recurrence or survival has been demonstrated between the two modalities, which allows decisions to focus on functional, esthetic, and psychological considerations.

Thus, while implant-based reconstruction remains a viable and sometimes necessary option, especially in thinner patients or those with comorbidities, autologous reconstruction is often regarded as the gold standard for long-term patient-reported outcomes, especially in younger or more active patients with high esthetic expectations.

6. Surgical decision-making and individualized planning

Modern breast reconstruction requires a patient centered approach that integrates oncologic context, anatomical characteristics, psychosocial factors, and esthetic goals into the surgical plan. Factors such as tumor stage, adjuvant therapy, body habits, comorbidities and patient preferences play a central role in defining reconstructive pathways. Factors such as tumor stage, adjuvant therapy, body habits, comorbidities, and patient preferences play a central role in defining reconstructive pathways.

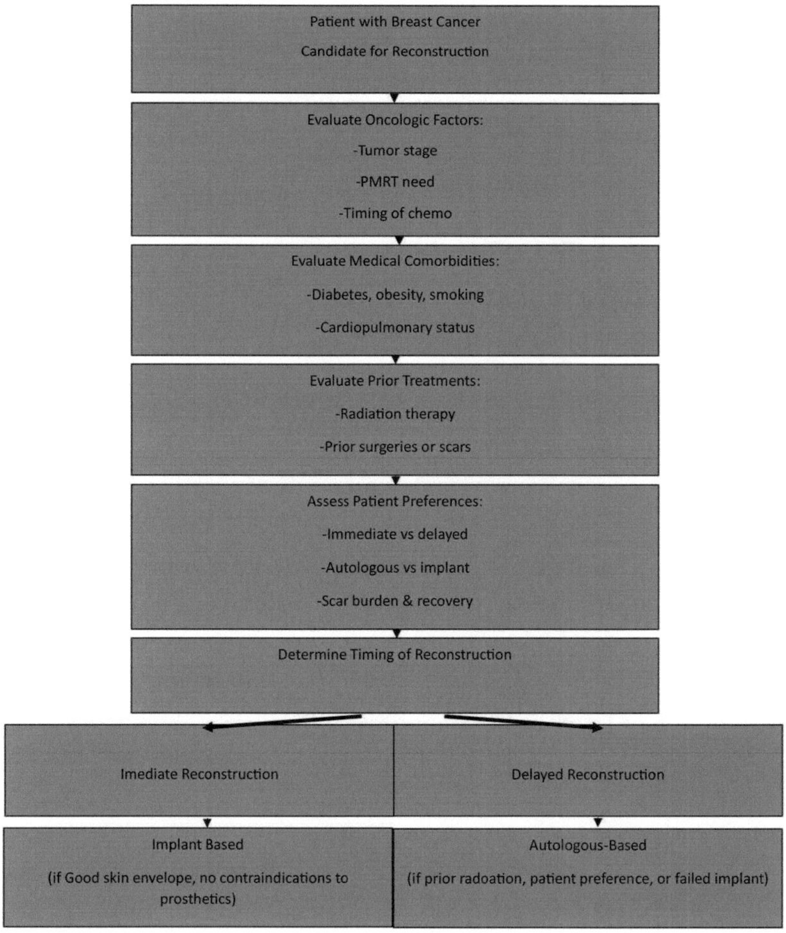

Figure 2.
Algorithm for technique selection.

6.1 Patient selection criteria

Proper patient selection is fundamental to optimizing outcomes in breast reconstruction. Surgical indication must be tailored based on oncologic status, medical comorbidities, anatomical considerations, prior treatments, and patient preferences as summarized in **Figure 2**.

6.2 Shared decision-making in multidisciplinary settings

Breast reconstruction occurs within a complex clinical landscape where shared decision making (SDM) has emerged as a cornerstone for delivering patient-centered care. In multidisciplinary breast cancer management, SDM involves collaborative dialog between the patient and a team that may include oncologists, plastic surgeons, breast surgeons, radiologists, pathologists, nurses, and psychologists.

Principles of Shared Decision-Making: [95].

1. Patient autonomy and engagement

   SDM respects patient values, preferences, and goals. Women facing breast reconstruction decisions must be fully informed about immediate vs. delayed reconstruction, implant-based vs. autologous techniques, potential complications, recovery time, and impact on oncologic treatment.

2. Balanced information exchange

   Clinicians provide evidence-based recommendations, while patients share their expectations and personal context. Tools such as decision aids, illustrations, and risk calculators (e.g., BREAST-Q, ACS Decision Tools) improve understanding and empowerment.

3. Integration of Multidisciplinary Input

   Coordinated input from multiple specialties ensures that the surgical plan aligns with:

   - Oncologic priorities (tumor biology, radiation/chemotherapy needs)
   - Medical safety (e.g., comorbidities, smoking, BMI)
   - Reconstructive feasibility (e.g., flap candidacy, donor site availability)

4. Documentation and Follow-Up

5. Decisions should be clearly documented with contingencies for treatment adaptations. Ongoing evaluation ensures alignment with evolving treatment stages or changes in patient status.

7. Global and resource-sensitive perspectives

7.1 Challenges in low-resource settings

Breast reconstruction after mastectomy remains a significant challenge in low resource settings due to limited access to specialized surgical teams, microsurgical infrastructure, and postoperative monitoring capabilities. In many developing regions, reconstructive options are often restricted by institutional capacity, economic constraints, and lack of trained personnel. These systematic limitations result in lower rates of reconstruction and limited surgical choice for patients. Additionally, the concentration of high complexity producers in urban tertiary centers further exacerbates geographic disparities in care. Therefore, adapting surgical strategies to the realities of local healthcare systems is crucial to expand reconstructive access globally.

7.2 Pedicled TRAM as a viable option in developing countries

The pedicled TRAM flap has reemerged as a valuable reconstructive method in resource limited environments. Its reliability, based on preserved vascular supply and minimal dependence on advanced technology, makes it suitable for smaller hospitals or community settings. Evidence from a community based study in the United States demonstrated favorable outcomes with low complication rates, no flap loss and positive patient satisfaction, despite limited resources [96].

The Technique also allows more surgeons to perform, especially those without microsurgical training, autologous reconstruction safely. In developing countries, the pedicled TRAM flap thus offers a feasible, effective, and scalable alternative that helps decentralize breast reconstruction services.

7.3 Cost-effectiveness and access to care

Economic considerations are pivotal when selecting reconstructive strategies in global health systems. In some countries a cost utility analysis comparing immediate and delayed reconstruction found both approaches to be financially sustainable for the national health system. Immediate reconstruction provided better quality adjusted life years with only a marginal increase in cost effectiveness [97].

Furthermore, while pedicled TRAM reconstructions may involve longer hospital stays or higher initial costs in some contexts, the absence of microsurgical demands and lower complication risks can translate into savings over time. Prioritizing cost efficient techniques such as the pedicled TRAM can improve access for underserved populations while maintaining satisfactory clinical outcomes.

8. Future directions and innovation

8.1 Advances in microsurgery and supermicrosurgery

In the last two decades, microsurgical breast reconstruction has evolved from a technically demanding option into a refined standard of care in high-volume centers. The advent of perforator flaps, particularly the deep inferior epigastric perforator (DIEP) flap, has significantly reduced donor site morbidity while preserving long-term esthetic outcomes [98].

Recent innovations in supermicrosurgery—defined as vascular anastomosis of vessels smaller than 0.8 mm-have opened new frontiers in flap—based reconstruction. Techniques like lymphaticovenular anastomosis (LVA) and vascularized lymph node transfer (VLNT) are now being integrated into breast reconstruction protocols to manage or prevent postmastectomy lymphedema, offering both functional and esthetic restoration in a single stage [99].

Technological advances such as robot-assisted microsurgery and fluorescence-guided anastomosis using indocyanine green (ICG) have enhanced precision and safety. Additionally, intraoperative microsurgical Doppler and thermal imaging are facilitating more reliable flap design, reducing fat necrosis and ischemia-related complications [100].

As training programs expand access to these techniques and surgical instrumentation becomes more refined, the microsurgical approach is poised to become the gold standard for complex breast reconstruction, particularly in young, active, and oncologically stable patients.

8.2 Role of 3D imaging and surgical planning software

Technological advances in three-dimensional (3D) imaging and virtual surgical planning (VSP) are transforming the field of breast reconstruction, enabling greater precision, personalization, and predictability of outcomes.

High-resolution 3D surface imaging systems allow for objective volumetric analysis, symmetry assessment, and preoperative planning. These tools enable surgeons to simulate expected outcomes, compare contralateral breast volume, and improve patient counseling by providing real-time visual models of proposed reconstructions [101].

Virtual surgical planning, particularly when integrated with computed tomography angiography (CTA), facilitates precise mapping of perforators for autologous flap harvest. This has led to significant reductions in operative time, intraoperative dissection, and flap-related complications [102].

Emerging AI-assisted platforms are being developed to analyze thousands of breast morphologies and surgical outcomes to predict optimal implant sizing or flap configuration. Combined with augmented reality (AR) tools and intraoperative navigation systems, the reconstruction process is moving toward a hybrid of art, data and precision engineering [103].

These technologies are also improving documentation and long-term monitoring of surgical results, opening the door for standardized outcome measurement across institutions and automated integrations with BREAST-Q data.

As accessibility increases, 3D imaging and planning software are expected to become routine elements in reconstructive practice, fostering a new era of digital surgical craftsmanship.

8.3 Tissue engineering and regenerative strategies

Tissue engineering and regenerative medicine are rapidly emerging as transformative forces in the future of breast reconstruction. The goal is to develop bioengineered solutions that mimic native tissue, reduce donor site morbidity and potentially eliminate the need for permanent implants.

One of the most promising avenues is the use of adipose-derived stem cells (ADSCs) in combination with scaffold-based constructs. These bioactive matrices, often made of collagen or polylactic acid, provide a 3D architecture that supports angiogenesis and adipogenesis, enabling the regeneration of soft tissue with more natural contour and feel [104].

Decellularized extracellular matrices (dECM), derived from porcine or human dermis, are also being investigated as scaffolds capable of inducing tissue-specific regeneration while minimizing immune rejection. These acellular bioscaffolds can be seeded with the patient's own cells or growth factors to accelerate integration and volume maintenance [105]. In parallel, 3D bioprinting technologies are under development to fabricate customized breast scaffolds with high anatomical fidelity. Although still in experimental stages, early studies suggest that layered constructs infused with vascular endothelial growth factor (VEGF) may support neovascularization and long-term tissue viability [106].

Moreover, fat grafting, once considered a purely esthetic adjunct, is now evolving into a regenerative therapy. When enriched with stromal vascular fraction (SVF) or platelet-rich plasma (PRP), autologous fat transfers show enhanced graft retention and skin quality improvements, particularly in irradiated fields [107]. The regenerative strategies hold immense potential to redefine the reconstructive paradigm, making breast restoration more biologically harmonious and less reliant on prosthetics or distant donor sites.

8.4 Addressing implant-related systemic symptoms

In recent years, increasing attention has been directed toward systemic symptoms reported by a subset of patients with breast implants-ranging from fatigue, arthralgia, cognitive dysfunction, to autoimmune-like phenomena. This clinical constellation has been informally referred to as "breast implant illness (BII)" and is partially encompassed by the broader concept of autoimmune/inflammatory Syndrome Induced by Adjuvants (ASIA) [108].

ASIA syndrome, first proposed by Shoenfeld in 2011, describes immune-mediated reactions to adjuvants such as silicone, mineral oils, and other biomaterials. While definitive causality between breast implants and systemic autoimmune diseases remains controversial, numerous case reports and patient advocacy groups have fueled interest in identifying biomarkers, diagnostic criteria, and standardized reporting protocols [109, 110].

Recent cohort studies suggest that a small percentage of patients may experience systematic symptoms that improve following explanation with or without bloc capsulectomy. However, the evidence remains low-level, primarily observational, and often lacks immunological confirmation [111].

From a reconstructive standpoint, patient selection, informed consent, and shared decision-making are critical. Surgeons must be equipped to discuss emerging data, offer alternatives (e.g., autologous reconstruction), and approach these patients with empathy rather than skepticism. Ongoing research is focused on the immunologic profile of susceptible patients, the role of biofilms, genetic predisposition, and development of "immnune-neutral" implant surface or fully reabsorbable scaffold materials [112].

In the context of rising demand for personalized and biologically safe reconstruction, addressing implant-related systemic symptoms represents both a clinical challenge and an ethical imperative for the next generation of plastic surgeons.

9. Conclusions

Reconstructive breast surgery has evolved into a highly specialized field, offering a broad spectrum of techniques that can be tailored to the individual patient's oncologic profile, anatomical considerations, and personal goals. Advances in microsurgery, implant technology, and biomaterials such as acellular dermal matrices have expanded reconstructive possibilities, enabling surgeons to achieve superior esthetic and functional outcomes.

Evidence synthesized from randomized trials, meta-analyses, and large-scale cohort studies underscores the importance of selecting the appropriate timing, technique, and reconstructive modality based on robust patient assessment. Autologous reconstruction, particularly with perforator flaps, consistently demonstrates higher long-term satisfaction and lower rates of implant-specific complications, while implant-based methods remain a valuable option for carefully selected candidates seeking shorter operative times and reduced donor-site morbidity.

Optimization of modifiable risk factors, including glycemic control in diabetic patients, weight management, and smoking cessation, is essential to reducing complication rates. In patients requiring postmastectomy radiation therapy, a delayed or staged reconstructive approach may preserve outcomes and minimize revision surgery.

Ultimately, the best reconstructive strategy emerges from a multidisciplinary, patient-centered decision-making process that incorporates oncologic safety, technical expertise, and long-term quality-of-life considerations. Continued research, particularly in the form of prospective multicenter trials and patient-reported outcome studies, will be critical in refining algorithms, reducing disparities in access, and further improving the standard of care in breast reconstruction.

Author details

Alba Mayra Padilla*, Celina Verónica Kishi, Heriberto Contreras,
Karla Elizabeth Rincón, Pablo Meneses and Maximiliano Sánchez
Jalisco Plastic and Reconstructive Surgery Institute "Dr. Jose Guerrerosantos",
Guadalajara, Mexico

*Address all correspondence to: mayrapadillamd@gmail.com

References

[1] Sung H, Ferlay J, Siegel RL, Laversanne M, Soerjomataram I, Jemal A, et al. Global cancer statistics 2020: GLOBOCAN estimates of incidence and mortality worldwide for 36 cancers in 185 countries. CA: A Cancer Journal for Clinicians. 2021;**71**(3):209-249

[2] Devi S. Projected global rise in breast cancer incidence and mortality by 2050. The Lancet Oncology. 2025;**26**(4):417

[3] Wilkins EG, Cederna PS, Lowery JC, Davis JA, Kim HM, Roth RS, et al. Prospective analysis of psychosocial outcomes in breast reconstruction: One-year postoperative results from the Michigan breast reconstruction outcome study. Plastic and Reconstructive Surgery. 2000;**106**(5):1014-1025; discussion 1026-7

[4] Atisha DM, Rushing CN, Samsa GP, Locklear TD, Cox CE, Shelley Hwang E, et al. A national snapshot of satisfaction with breast cancer procedures. Annals of Surgical Oncology. 2015;**22**(2):361-369

[5] Pusic AL, Klassen AF, Scott AM, Klok JA, Cordeiro PG, Cano SJ. Development of a new patient-reported outcome measure for breast surgery: The BREAST-Q. Plastic and Reconstructive Surgery. 2009;**124**(2):345-353

[6] Uroskie TW, Colen LB. History of breast reconstruction. Seminars in Plastic Surgery. 2004;**18**(2):65-69

[7] Spear SL, Onyewu C. Staged breast reconstruction with saline-filled implants in the irradiated breast: Recent trends and therapeutic implications. Plastic and Reconstructive Surgery. 2000;**105**(3):930-942

[8] Pumilia A, Le PB, Bian J, Becker ME, Friedman HI. Implant-based breast reconstruction—A systematic review and meta-analysis of prepectoral versus submuscular implant placement. Annals of Breast Surgery. 2025;**9**:11

[9] Blondeel N, Vanderstraeten GG, Monstrey SJ, Van Landuyt K, Tonnard P, Lysens R, et al. The donor site morbidity of free DIEP flaps and free TRAM flaps for breast reconstruction. British Journal of Plastic Surgery. 1997;**50**(5):322-330

[10] Bajaj AK, Kon PS, Oberg KC, Miles DAG. Aesthetic outcomes in patients undergoing breast conservation therapy for the treatment of localized breast cancer. Plastic and Reconstructive Surgery. 2004;**114**(6):1442-1449

[11] Saour S, Libondi G, Ramakrishnan V. Microsurgical refinements with the use of internal mammary (IM) perforators as recipient vessels in transverse upper gracilis (TUG) autologous breast reconstruction. Gland Surgery. 2017;**6**(4):375-379

[12] Ydo CB, Lilja C, Naseri S, Sørensen JA, Thomsen JB. A standardized preoperative imaging regime reduces major complications in abdominal free flaps breast reconstruction– A retrospective cohort study. European Journal of Plastic Surgery. 2025;**48**(1):4. DOI: 10.1007/s00238-025-02314-5

[13] Teunis T, Heerma van Voss MR, Kon M, van Maurik JFMM. CT-angiography prior to DIEP flap breast reconstruction: A systematic review and meta-analysis. Microsurgery. 2013;**33**(6):496-502

[14] Beugels J, Bijkerk E, Lataster A, Heuts EM, van der Hulst RRWJ, Tuinder SMH. Nerve coaptation improves the sensory recovery of the breast in DIEP flap breast reconstruction. Plastic and Reconstructive Surgery. 2021;**148**(2):273-284

[15] Offodile AC 2nd, Gu C, Boukovalas S, Coroneos CJ, Chatterjee A, Largo RD, et al. Enhanced recovery after surgery (ERAS) pathways in breast reconstruction: Systematic review and meta-analysis of the literature. Breast Cancer Research and Treatment. 2019;**173**(1):65-77

[16] Stefura T, Rusinek J, Wator J, Zagórski A, Zając M, Libondi G, et al. Implant vs. autologous tissue-based breast reconstruction: A systematic review and meta-analysis of the studies comparing surgical approaches in 55,455 patients. Journal of Plastic, Reconstructive & Aesthetic Surgery. 2023;77:346-358. DOI: 10.1016/j.bjps.2022.11.044

[17] Chinese Society of Breast Surgery (CSBrS). Clinical practice guideline for postmastectomy breast reconstruction (2021 edition). Chinese Medical Journal. 2021;**134**(19):2272-2274

[18] Saldanha J, Broyles JM, Lee E. Outcomes of implant-based breast reconstruction after mastectomy for breast cancer: A systematic review and meta-analysis. Journal of Plastic, Reconstructive & Aesthetic Surgery. 2022;**75**(10):3784-3793

[19] Saldanha IJ, Broyles JM, Adam GP, Cao W, Bhuma MR, Mehta S, et al. Autologous breast reconstruction after mastectomy for breast cancer: A systematic review. Plastic and Reconstructive Surgery – Global Open. 2022;**10**(3):e4181. DOI: 10.1097/GOX.0000000000004181

[20] Yun JH, Diaz R, Orman AG. Breast reconstruction and radiation therapy. Cancer Control. 2018;**25**(1):1073274818795489

[21] Santosa KB, Qi J, Kim HM, Hamill JB, Wilkins EG, Pusic AL. Long-term patient-reported outcomes in postmastectomy breast reconstruction. JAMA Surgery. 2018;**153**(10):891-899

[22] Awadeen A, Fareed M, Elameen AM. The impact of postmastectomy radiotherapy on the outcomes of prepectoral implant-based breast reconstruction: A systematic review and meta-analysis. Aesthetic Plastic Surgery. 2023;**47**(1):81-91

[23] Sbitany H, Piper M, Lentz R. Prepectoral breast reconstruction: A safe alternative to submuscular prosthetic reconstruction following nipple-sparing mastectomy. Plastic and Reconstructive Surgery. 2017;**140**(3):432-443. DOI: 10.1097/PRS.0000000000003627

[24] Ostapenko E, Nixdorf L, Devyatko Y, Exner R, Wimmer K, Fitzal F. Prepectoral versus subpectoral implant-based breast reconstruction: A systematic review and meta-analysis. Annals of Surgical Oncology. 2023;**30**(1):126-136. Epub 2022 Oct 16. DOI: 10.1245/s10434-022-12567-0

[25] Arnautovic A, Karinja S, Olafsson S, Carty MJ, Erdmann-Sager J, Caterson SA, et al. Optimal timing of delayed microvascular breast reconstruction after radiation therapy. Journal of Reconstructive Microsurgery. 2023;**39**(3):165-170. DOI: 10.1055/s-0042-1750125

[26] Cordeiro PG, Pusic AL, Disa JJ. Irradiation after immediate tissue expander/implant breast reconstruction: Outcomes, complications, aesthetic results, and satisfaction among

156 patients. Plastic and Reconstructive Surgery. 2015;**135**(6):1454-1463

[27] Mureau MAM, Breast Reconstruction Guideline Working Group. Dutch breast reconstruction guideline. Journal of Plastic, Reconstructive & Aesthetic Surgery. 2018;**71**(3):290-304. DOI: 10.1016/j.bjps.2017.12.020. Epub 2017 Dec 27

[28] Margulies IG, Salzberg CA. The use of acellular dermal matrix in breast reconstruction: Evolution of techniques over 2 decades. Gland Surgery. 2019;**8**(1):3-10. DOI: 10.21037/gs.2018.10.05

[29] Elameen AM, AlMarakby MA, Atta TI, Dahy AA. The risk of breast implant-associated anaplastic large cell lymphoma; a systematic review and meta-analysis. Aesthetic Plastic Surgery. 2024;**48**(24):5315-5328. DOI: 10.1007/s00266-024-03956-9. Epub 2024 May 9

[30] Turin SY, Gutowski K. Bioabsorbable polydioxanone mesh for soft tissue reinforcement in revisional breast surgery. Aesthetic Surgery Journal. Open Forum. 2022;**4**:ojac004

[31] Becker H. Update on the use of synthetic mesh in reconstructive and cosmetic breast surgery. Aesthetic Plastic Surgery. 2020;**44**(4):1128-1129

[32] Sweitzer K, Arias-Camison R, Cafro C, Langstein H. The use of reinforced ovine mesh in implant breast reconstruction: Equivalent outcomes to human acellular dermal matrices and more cost-effective. Annals of Plastic Surgery. 2024;**93**(6):664-667

[33] Haddock NT, Facchin F, Teotia SS. A clinical practice review on process efficiency in autologous breast reconstruction. Gland Surgery. 2023;**12**(7):1007-1015

[34] Edsander-Nord A, Jurell G, Wickman M. Donor-site morbidity after pedicled or free TRAM flap surgery: A prospective and objective study. Plastic and Reconstructive Surgery. 1998;**102**(5):1508-1516

[35] Chevray PM. Update on breast reconstruction using free TRAM, DIEP, and SIEA flaps. Seminars in Plastic Surgery. 2004;**18**(2):97-104

[36] Garvey PB, Buchel EW, Pockaj BA, Casey WJ 3rd, Gray RJ, Hernández JL, et al. DIEP and pedicled TRAM flaps: A comparison of outcomes. Plastic and Reconstructive Surgery. 2006;**117**(6):1711-1719; discussion 1720-1

[37] Schwitzer JA, Miller HC, Pusic AL, Matros E, Mehrara BJ, McCarthy CM, et al. Satisfaction following unilateral breast reconstruction: A comparison of pedicled TRAM and free abdominal flaps. Plastic and Reconstructive Surgery. Global Open. 2015;**3**(8):e482

[38] Lee WS, Park SO, Kim IK. Prevention of abdominal bulging using onlay dermal autografts from discarded zone IV TRAM flap tissue. Journal of Clinical Medicine. 2022;**11**(7):1929

[39] Butler PD, Wu LC. Abdominal perforator vs. muscle sparing flaps for breast reconstruction. Gland Surgery. 2015;**4**(3):212-221

[40] Egeberg A, Rasmussen MK, Sørensen JA. Comparing the donor-site morbidity using DIEP, SIEA or MS-TRAM flaps for breast reconstructive surgery: A meta-analysis. Journal of Plastic, Reconstructive & Aesthetic Surgery. 2012;**65**(11):1474-1480

[41] Nelissen SH, Krijnen NA, Tsehaie J, Schellekens PPA, Paes EC, Simmermacher RKJ, et al. Bulging after DIEP breast reconstruction:

New insights concerning rectus diastasis and medial perforator harvest. Plastic and Reconstructive Surgery. Global Open. 2023;**11**(3):e4840

[42] Haddock NT, Culver AJ, Teotia SS. Abdominal weakness, bulge, or hernia after DIEP flaps: An algorithm of management, prevention, and surgical repair with classification. Journal of Plastic, Reconstructive & Aesthetic Surgery. 2021;**74**(9):2194-2201

[43] Wu LC, Bajaj A, Chang DW, Chevray PM. Comparison of donor-site morbidity of SIEA, DIEP, and muscle-sparing TRAM flaps for breast reconstruction. Plastic and Reconstructive Surgery. 2008;**122**(3):702-709

[44] Coroneos CJ, Heller AM, Voineskos SH, Avram R. SIEA versus DIEP arterial complications: A cohort study. Plastic and Reconstructive Surgery. 2015;**135**(5):802e-807e

[45] Somers S, Foley B, Dadzie A, Hart C, Chen J, Bautista CH, et al. A comparison of SIEA/SCIA and DIEP flaps for autologous breast reconstruction. Journal of Reconstructive Microsurgery. 2025;**42**:7-15. DOI: 10.1055/a-2540-0987

[46] Banys-Paluchowski M, Brus L, Krawczyk N, Kopperschmidt SV, Gasparri ML, Bündgen N, et al. Latissimus dorsi flap for breast reconstruction: A large single-institution evaluation of surgical outcome and complications. Archives of Gynecology and Obstetrics. 2024;**309**(1):269-280

[47] Haddad Tame JL, Jiménez Muñoz Ledo G. Anatomical and surgical description of a new concept in breast reconstruction: Muscle sparing dorsoepigastric flap of latissimus dorsi. Cirugía Plástica Ibero-Latinoamericana. 2012;**38**(1):27-34

[48] Højvig JH, Henriksen M, Bartholdy CR, Bonde CT. Donor-site morbidity following breast reconstruction with a latissimus dorsi flap - A prospective study. Journal of Plastic, Reconstructive & Aesthetic Surgery. 2022;**75**(7):2205-2210

[49] Homsy C, Theunissen T, Sadeghi A. The thoracodorsal artery perforator flap: A powerful tool in breast reconstruction. Plastic Reconstructive Surgery [Internet]. 2022;**150**(4):755-761. DOI: 10.1097/PRS.0000000000009576

[50] Maier MA, Hoffman RD, Kordahi AM, Levine J, Hilaire H St., Allen RJ Sr. Surgical delay of thoracodorsal artery perforator flaps for total autologous breast reconstruction. Annals of Plastic Surgery. 2024;**92**(2):161-168

[51] Haddock NT, Gassman A, Cho MJ, Teotia SS. 101 consecutive profunda artery perforator flaps in breast reconstruction: Lessons learned with our early experience. Plastic and Reconstructive Surgery. 2017;**140**(2):229-239

[52] Atzeni M, Salzillo R, Haywood R, Persichetti P, Figus A. Breast reconstruction using the profunda artery perforator (PAP) flap: Technical refinements and evolution, outcomes, and patient satisfaction based on 116 consecutive flaps. Journal of Plastic, Reconstructive & Aesthetic Surgery. 2022;**75**(5):1617-1624

[53] Fosseprez P, Gerdom A, Servaes M, Deconinck C, Pirson G, Berners A. Profunda artery perforator flap: Reliable secondary option for breast reconstruction? Annales de Chirurgie Plastique et Esthétique. 2017;**62**(6):637-645

[54] Largo RD, Chu CK, Chang EI, Liu J, Abu-Ghname A, Wang H, et al. Perforator mapping of the profunda artery perforator flap: Anatomy and clinical experience: Anatomy and clinical experience. Plastic and Reconstructive Surgery. 2020;**146**(5):1135-1145

[55] Cohen Z, Azoury SC, Nelson JA, Haglich K, Dayan JH, Matros E, et al. The preferred design of the profunda artery perforator flap for autologous breast reconstruction: Transverse or diagonal? Plastic and Reconstructive Surgery. Global Open. 2023;**11**(8):e5188

[56] Qian B, Xiong L, Li J, Sun Y, Sun J, Guo N, et al. A systematic review and meta-analysis on microsurgical safety and efficacy of profunda artery perforator flap in breast reconstruction. Journal of Oncology. 2019;**2019**:9506720

[57] Buntic RF, Horton KM, Brooks D, Althubaiti GA. Transverse upper gracilis flap as an alternative to abdominal tissue breast reconstruction: Technique and modifications: Technique and modifications. Plastic and Reconstructive Surgery. 2011;**128**(6):607e-613e

[58] Park JE, Alkureishi LWT, Song DH. TUGs into VUGs and friendly BUGs: Transforming the gracilis territory into the best secondary breast reconstructive option. Plastic and Reconstructive Surgery. 2015;**136**(3):447-454

[59] Craggs B, Vanmierlo B, Zeltzer A, Buyl R, Haentjens P, Hamdi M. Donor-site morbidity following harvest of the transverse myocutaneous gracilis flap for breast reconstruction. Plastic and Reconstructive Surgery. 2014;**134**(5):682e-691e

[60] Hunter JE, Lardi AM, Dower DR, Farhadi J. Evolution from the TUG to PAP flap for breast reconstruction: Comparison and refinements of technique. Journal of Plastic, Reconstructive & Aesthetic Surgery. 2015;**68**(7):960-965

[61] Murphy DC, Razzano S, Wade RG, Haywood RM, Figus A. Inferior gluteal artery perforator (IGAP) flap versus profunda artery perforator (PAP) flap as an alternative option for free autologous breast reconstruction. Journal of Plastic, Reconstructive & Aesthetic Surgery. 2022;**75**(3):1100-1107

[62] LoTempio MM, Allen RJ. Breast reconstruction with SGAP and IGAP flaps. Plastic and Reconstructive Surgery. 2010;**126**(2):393-401

[63] Martineau J, Scampa M, Viscardi JA, Giordano S, Kalbermatten DF, Oranges CM. Inferior gluteal artery perforator (IGAP) flap in autologous breast reconstruction: A proportional meta-analysis of surgical outcomes. Journal of Plastic, Reconstructive & Aesthetic Surgery. 2023;**84**:147-156

[64] Tuinder SMH, Beugels J, Lataster A, de Haan MW, Piatkowski A, Saint-Cyr M, et al. The lateral thigh perforator flap for autologous breast reconstruction: A prospective analysis of 138 flaps. Plastic and Reconstructive Surgery. 2018;**141**(2):257-268

[65] Tessler O, Guste J, Bartow MJ, Torabi R, Gimenez A, Patel SB, et al. Stacked lateral thigh perforator flap as a novel option for autologous breast reconstruction. Plastic and Reconstructive Surgery. 2019;**143**(6):1601-1604

[66] Stillaert FBJL, Opsomer D, Blondeel PN, Van Landuyt K. The lumbar artery perforator flap in breast reconstruction. Plastic and Reconstructive Surgery. 2023;**151**(1):41-44

[67] Fisher MH, Greenspun DT. Lumbar artery perforator free flaps for breast reconstruction. Plastic and Aesthetic Research. 2024;**11**:11-36. DOI: 10.20517/2347-9264.2024.53

[68] Haddock NT, Teotia SS. Lumbar artery perforator flap: Initial experience with simultaneous bilateral flaps for breast reconstruction. Plastic and Reconstructive Surgery. Global Open. 2020;**8**(5):e2800

[69] Bordianu A, Leoveanu I, Chang EI. Autologous breast reconstruction beyond the DIEP: A narrative review of autologous breast reconstruction options beyond the DIEP flap. Annals of Breast Surgery. 2020;**4**:15. DOI: 10.21037/abs-20-66

[70] Sun Y, Liu Q, Zhu J, Hu H, Lu L, Ying J, et al. Optimal strategies for autologous fat grafting in breast augmentation and reconstruction: A systematic review and network meta-analysis. Plastic and Reconstructive Surgery [Internet]. 2024;**155**(2):2-10. DOI: 10.1097/PRS.0000000000011653

[71] Navarro AS, Omalek D, Chaltiel L, Vaysse C, Meresse T, Gangloff D, et al. Oncologic safety of autologous fat grafting in primary breast reconstruction after mastectomy for cancer. European Journal of Surgical Oncology. 2024;**50**(4):107998

[72] Chen J, Alghamdi AA, Wong CY, Alnaim MF, Kuper G, Zhang J. The efficacy of fat grafting on treating post-mastectomy pain with and without breast reconstruction: A systematic review and meta-analysis. Current Oncology. 2024;**31**(4):2057-2066

[73] Yesantharao PS, Nguyen DH. Hybrid breast reconstruction: A systematic review of current trends and future directions. Annals of Breast Surgery. 2022;**6**:17-17

[74] Jiménez Muñoz-Ledo G, Sosa Vázquez A, Cueva Rubio JA, Olvera Zambrano CA, Torres Gómez B, Padilla Correa AM, et al. Concepto de marco mamario y su manejo: optimizando el resultado estético. Cirugia plástica ibero-latinoamericana. 2025;**51**(1):9-18

[75] Jimenez Muñoz Ledo G, Ortiz H, Padilla AM. Anatomic areas of lipoframing in breast surgery. Cureus. 2024;**16**(3):e57216

[76] Wu Young MY, Garza RM, Chang DW. Immediate versus delayed autologous breast reconstruction in patients undergoing post-mastectomy radiation therapy: A paradigm shift. Journal of Surgical Oncology. 2022;**126**(6):949-955

[77] Parmeshwar N, Barnes L, Martins D, Nicholas C, Piper M. The impact of post-mastectomy radiation timing on overall outcomes of autologous free-flap breast reconstruction. Microsurgery. 2024;**44**(1):e31091

[78] Pruimboom T, Schols RM, Van Kuijk SMJ, Van der Hulst RR, Qiu SS. Indocyanine green angiography for preventing postoperative mastectomy skin flap necrosis in immediate breast reconstruction. The Cochrane Library [Internet]. 2020;**2020**(4):4-43. DOI: 10.1002/14651858.cd013280.pub2

[79] Toyoda Y, Fu RH, Li L, Otterburn DM, Rohde CH. Smoking as an independent risk factor for postoperative complications in plastic surgical procedures: A propensity score–matched analysis of 36,454 patients from the NSQIP database from 2005 to 2014. Plastic and Reconstructive Surgery. 2018;**141**(1):226-236

[80] De Lorenzi F, Gazzola R, Sangalli C, Villa O, Marchetti M, Monturano M, et al. Poly implant prothèse asymmetrical

anatomical breast implants: A product recall study. Plastic and Reconstructive Surgery. 2015;**135**(1):25-33

[81] Mortada H, Alwadai A, Bamakhrama B, Alsinan T, Hanawi MD, Alfaryan SM, et al. The impact of diabetes mellitus on breast reconstruction outcomes and complications: A systematic literature review and meta-analysis. Aesthetic Plastic Surgery. 2023;**47**(2):570-583

[82] Kufel-Grabowska J, Podolak A, Maliszewski D, Bartoszkiewicz M, Ramlau R, Lukaszuk K. Fertility counseling in BRCA1/2-mutated women with breast cancer and healthy individuals. Journal of Clinical Medicine. 2022;**11**(14):3996

[83] Ramos-Gallardo G, Herrán-Motta FS, Bustamante-Lambaren LA, Kishi-Sutto CV, Sánchez-Vanegas M, Robledo-Madrid P, et al. Seguridad en reconstrucción mamaria. Medicina basada en evidencias. Recomendaciones. Cirugía Plástica. 2024;**34**(4):140-146

[84] Isaac KV, Buchel EW, Brackstone MM, Doherty C, Lipa JE, Zhong T, et al. Canadian expert opinion on breast reconstruction access: Strategies to optimize care during COVID-19. Plastic and Reconstructive Surgery. Global Open. 2022;**10**(2):e4204

[85] Chang DW, Wang B, Robb GL, Reece GP, Miller MJ, Evans GR, et al. Effect of obesity on flap and donor-site complications in free transverse rectus abdominis myocutaneous flap breast reconstruction. Plastic and Reconstructive Surgery. 2000;**105**(5):1640-1648

[86] Rawan RA, Prabhu N, Alibrahim A. Autologous versus alloplastic reconstruction for patients with obesity: A systematic review and meta-analysis. Aesthetic Plastic Surgery. 2022;**46**(3):597-609

[87] Goltsman D, Munabi N, Ascherman JA. The association between smoking and complications in plastic surgery: A systematic review and meta-analysis. Plastic and Reconstructive Surgery. 2017;**139**(2):503-511

[88] Jouve E, Giordano-Labadie F, Selmes G, Soule-Tholy M, Navarro AS, Gangloff D, et al. Delayed hypersensitivity reaction to titanium-coated polypropylene mesh in breast reconstruction. Plastic and Reconstructive Surgery. Global Open. 2022;**10**(4):e4232

[89] Nguyen J, Popovic M, Chow E, Cella D, Beaumont JL, Chu D, et al. EORTC QLQ-BR23 and FACT-B for the assessment of quality of life in patients with breast cancer: A literature review. Journal of Comparative Effectiveness Research. 2015;**4**(2):157-166

[90] Metcalfe KA, Semple J, Quan ML, Vadaparampil ST, Holloway C, Brown M, et al. Changes in psychosocial functioning 1 year after mastectomy alone, delayed breast reconstruction, or immediate breast reconstruction. Annals of Surgical Oncology. 2012;**19**(1):233-241

[91] Tsantakis V, Dimitroulis DA, Kontzoglou KC, Nikiteas NI. Investigating the difference in quality of life between immediate and delayed breast cancer reconstruction: A systematic review. Cancer Diagnosis & Prognosis. 2024;**4**(3):223-230

[92] Eltahir Y, Werners LLCH, Dreise MM, van Emmichoven IAZ, Jansen L, Werker PMN, et al. Quality-of-life outcomes between mastectomy alone and breast reconstruction: Comparison of patient-reported BREAST-Q and other health-related quality-of-life measures.

Plastic and Reconstructive Surgery. 2013;**132**(2):201e-209e

[93] Ng SK, Hare RM, Kuang RJ, Smith KM, Brown BJ, Hunter-Smith DJ. Breast reconstruction post mastectomy: Patient satisfaction and decision making. Annals of Plastic Surgery. 2016;**76**(6):640-644

[94] Jagsi R, Jiang J, Momoh AO, Alderman A, Giordano SH, Buchholz TA, et al. Complications after mastectomy and immediate breast reconstruction for breast cancer: A claims-based analysis: A claims-based analysis. Annals of Surgery. 2016;**263**(2):219-227

[95] Cordeiro PG. Breast reconstruction after surgery for breast cancer. The New England Journal of Medicine. 2008;**359**(15):1590-1601

[96] Long Z, Huettner F, Kells A. Pedicled myocutaneous flap breast reconstruction in the community hospital setting: An analysis of cost and complications. Cureus. 2020;**12**(11):e11806

[97] Perea AH, Rosselli D. Análisis de costo-utilidad en Colombia del tratamiento integral del carcinoma de seno con reconstrucción inmediata frente a la reconstrucción diferida. Biomédica. 2018;**38**(3):363-378

[98] Santanelli F, Longo B, Angelini M, Laporta R, Paolini G. Prospective computerized analyses of sensibility in breast reconstruction with non-reinnervated DIEP flap. Plastic and Reconstructive Surgery. 2011;**127**(5):1790-1795

[99] Schaverien MV, Badash I, Patel KM, Selber JC, Cheng MH. Vascularized lymph node transfer for lymphedema. Seminars in Plastic Surgery. 2018;**32**(1):28-35

[100] Nassar AH, Maselli AM, Manstein S, Shiah E, Slatnick BL, Dowlatshahi AS, et al. Comparison of various modalities utilized for preoperative planning in microsurgical reconstructive surgery. Journal of Reconstructive Microsurgery. 2022;**38**(3):170-180

[101] Losken A, Seify H, Denson DD, Paredes AA Jr, Carlson GW. Validating three-dimensional imaging of the breast. Annals of Plastic Surgery. 2005;**54**(5):471-476; discussion 477-8

[102] Rozen WM, Ashton MW, Stella DL, Phillips TJ, Grinsell D, Taylor GI. The accuracy of computed tomographic angiography for mapping the perforators of the deep inferior epigastric artery: A blinded, prospective cohort study. Plastic and Reconstructive Surgery. 2008;**122**(4):1003-1009

[103] Gouveia PF, Luna R, Fontes F, Pinto D, Mavioso C, Anacleto J, et al. Augmented reality in breast surgery education. Breast Care (Basel). 2023;**18**(3):182-186

[104] Kim YJ, Jeong JH. Clinical application of adipose stem cells in plastic surgery. Journal of Korean Medical Science. 2014;**29**(4):462-467

[105] Flynn LE. The use of decellularized adipose tissue to provide an inductive microenvironment for the adipogenic differentiation of human adipose-derived stem cells. Biomaterials. 2010;**31**(17):4715-4724

[106] Chhaya MP, Melchels FPW, Holzapfel BM, Baldwin JG, Hutmacher DW. Sustained regeneration of high-volume adipose tissue for breast reconstruction using computer aided design and biomanufacturing. Biomaterials. 2015;**52**:551-560

[107] Turner A, Abu-Ghname A, Davis MJ, Winocour SJ, Hanson SE, Chu CK. Fat grafting in breast reconstruction. Seminars in Plastic Surgery. 2020;**34**(1):17-23

[108] Shoenfeld Y, Agmon-Levin N. "ASIA" - Autoimmune/inflammatory syndrome induced by adjuvants. Journal of Autoimmunity. 2011;**36**(1):4-8

[109] Watad A, Sharif K, Shoenfeld Y. The ASIA syndrome: Basic concepts. Mediterranean Journal of Rheumatology. 2017;**28**(2):64-69

[110] de Boer M, Colaris M, van der Hulst RRWJ, Cohen Tervaert JW. Is explantation of silicone breast implants useful in patients with complaints? Immunologic Research. 2017;**65**(1):25-36

[111] Magnusson MR, Cooter RD, Rakhorst H, McGuire PA, Adams WP Jr, Deva AK. Breast implant illness: A way forward. Plastic and Reconstructive Surgery. 2019;**143**(3S A Review of Breast Implant-Associated Anaplastic Large Cell Lymphoma):74S-81S

[112] Foroushani FT, Dzobo K, Khumalo NP, Mora VZ, de Mezerville R, Bayat A. Advances in surface modifications of the silicone breast implant and impact on its biocompatibility and biointegration. Biomaterials Research. 2022;**26**(1):80

Chapter 3

A Structured Approach to DIEP Flap Reconstruction: Imaging, Execution, and Handling Surgical Challenges

Samarth Gupta and Venkat Ramakrishnan

Abstract

We present a structured, stepwise approach to deep inferior epigastric artery perforator (DIEP) flap breast reconstruction that integrates high-resolution computed tomographic angiography (CTA) and refined intraoperative techniques. Preoperative CTA mapping of abdominal perforators and venous drainage provides a detailed vascular roadmap, assisting in operative planning and highlighting the patient-specific anatomical variations. This imaging-driven planning facilitates algorithmic intraoperative decision-making for optimal perforator selection. This allows surgeons to correlate CTA data with surface anatomy, enabling precise perforator localization. These measures shorten flap dissection time, resulting in more efficient flap harvests and potentially reduced complications. Selective venous supercharging is employed in flaps at risk of venous congestion and cases with a dominant superficial venous system. In these situations, an additional anastomosis of the superficial inferior epigastric vein (SIEV) provides augmented outflow and can avert postoperative congestion. Finally, our approach addresses complex scenarios requiring greater tissue volume. For extensive chest wall defects, a bipedicled DIEP flap can be utilized to harvest the entire lower abdominal skin-fat flap, ensuring adequate perfusion across a broad area. Preoperative CTA is indispensable in these cases for mapping both pedicles and guiding anastomotic configurations that maximize perfusion overlap. This structured approach—combining advanced imaging with algorithmic surgical strategies—aims to improve the safety, efficiency, and versatility of DIEP flap reconstruction.

Keywords: DIEP flap, CTA-guided planning, perforator selection, venous supercharging, reconstructive microsurgery

1. Introduction

The deep inferior epigastric perforator (DIEP) flap represents the culmination of decades of evolution in abdominal-based autologous breast reconstruction. Earlier techniques like the pedicled and free TRAM flaps (transverse rectus abdominis myocutaneous flaps) were pioneering in the 1980s but required sacrificing some or all of the rectus

IntechOpen

abdominis muscle [1]. The DIEP flap, first described in 1989, marked a major advancement by preserving the abdominal muscle and utilizing only skin and fat perfused by perforating vessels of the deep inferior epigastric system [1, 2]. The core strategy of the DIEP technique has remained to harvest the lower abdominal adipocutaneous tissue while retaining the continuity, innervation, and function of the rectus muscle, yielding excellent breast shape and abdominal wall integrity [3]. Over time, the DIEP flap has become *the preferred autologous option* for many patients, offering a "natural" reconstruction that can last a lifetime with minimal long-term morbidity at the donor site [4].

Despite its advantages, the DIEP flap introduces unique challenges that necessitate a meticulous and structured approach. Early DIEP surgeons often relied on extensive intraoperative exploration to find the suitable perforators, which could prolong surgery and increase complexity. Moreover, the microsurgical skill required to anastomose these delicate vessels is considerable—these operations have a steep learning curve for trainees and junior surgeons [5]. Operating time and re-exploration rates do improve with experience, but achieving consistency in outcomes demands careful planning and technique. In the absence of a structured plan, surgeons may face higher risks of venous congestion and partial flap necrosis, and the technical demands can lead to prolonged ischemia times or errors in less experienced hands. Recognizing these challenges, modern reconstructive teams have sought strategies to make DIEP flap surgery more predictable and reproducible. In this chapter, we will provide an overview of the history, relevant anatomy, imaging techniques, intraoperative perforator selection, and strategies for managing complex cases, with the aim of achieving optimal outcomes in breast reconstruction.

2. Brief history of the evolution of the DIEP flap

The foundation for abdominal-based flap reconstruction was laid in the late 1970s, beginning with Holmström's description of the "free abdominoplasty flap" in 1979 [6]. This pioneering concept introduced the idea of microsurgically transferring abdominal tissue, marking a significant departure from pedicled flap designs. In 1982,

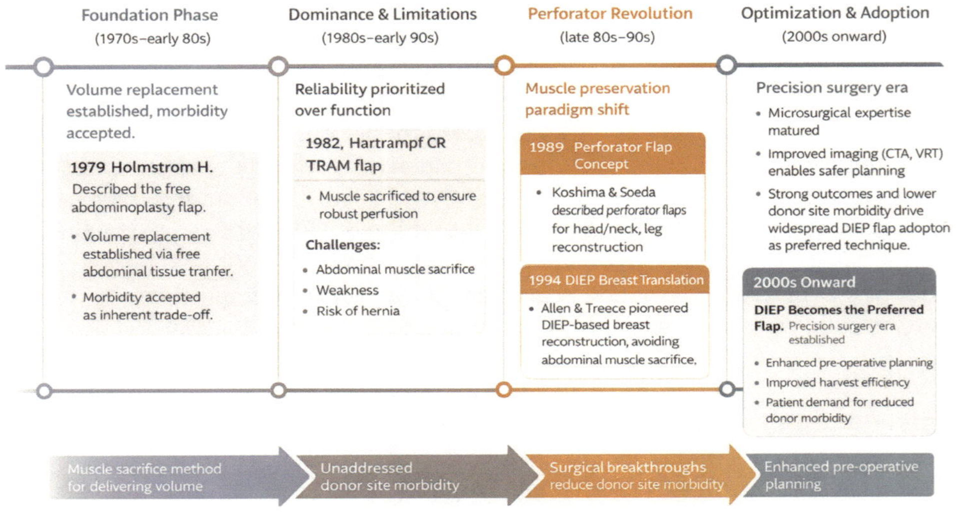

Figure 1.
Timeline showing key milestones in the evolution of the DIEP flap from early abdominal flaps (TRAM) to modern DIEP flap.

Hartrampf et al. popularized the pedicled TRAM (transverse rectus abdominis myocutaneous) flap, which retained part of the rectus muscle but brought enhanced reliability and volume for breast reconstruction [7].

Allen and Treece published the first report on the DIEP flap in 1994, emphasizing muscle preservation and improved functional outcomes [8]. However, it was Dr. Venkat Ramakrishnan, the senior author of this chapter, who performed one of the earliest DIEP flap reconstructions prior to this publication. His contribution represents a landmark moment in the clinical application of this technique in the UK, marking the beginning of widespread DIEP flap adoption in Europe [9]. Subsequent prospective studies, such as Blondeel's 1998 series of 100 DIEP flaps, validated the technique's safety and advantages over TRAM flaps, cementing the DIEP flap as the gold standard in autologous breast reconstruction today (**Figure 1**) [8, 10].

3. Applied anatomy, pre-operative imaging, and flap planning

3.1 Abdominal flap perfusion anatomy

Classically, the perfusion of a transverse lower abdominal flap (such as a TRAM or DIEP flap) was described in terms of four perfusion zones. This concept originated from Scheflan and Dinner's work in 1983 and was popularized by Hartrampf et al. in 1990 [7]. In the traditional model, if the flap is supplied by the central pedicle, the territories are divided as: Zone I—the ipsilateral half of the flap (centered on the pedicle) which is most perfused; Zone II—the contralateral half *medial* portion (across the midline from Zone I); Zone III—the ipsilateral *lateral* portion; and Zone IV—the contralateral lateral edge, which is farthest from the blood supply [11]. Zone I has the highest perfusion, whereas Zone IV is the least perfused and most prone to ischemia (often discarded in practice).

However, subsequent research demonstrated that perfusion patterns are not fixed and can vary with the source of the blood supply. Scheflan and Dinner themselves noted that an ipsilateral lateral area often had better perfusion than the contralateral medial side, suggesting that *Zone III might be more vascularized than Zone II* in many cases [12]. In 2006, Holm et al. revisited perfusion zones using intraoperative fluorescent dye (ICG) imaging and confirmed that in DIEP flaps the ipsilateral lateral territory (original Zone III) can outperform the contralateral territory (Zone II). This effectively reversed zones II and III for planning purposes when a single perforator is used on one side.

Saint-Cyr et al. [13] and Rozen et al. [14] introduced the concept of the "perforasome"—the vascular territory of a single perforator—and demonstrated through 3D CT angiography and cadaver injections that medial-row perforators and lateral-row perforators have distinct perfusion footprints [13]. Medial row perforators (located near the umbilicus) tend to be larger and have a more central trajectory. They frequently cross the midline to supply the opposite hemiabdomen—in fact, one study found ~98% of medial perforators sent branches across the midline [14]. Thus, a flap based on a robust medial perforator can often perfuse the contralateral half (old Zone II) quite well. Lateral row perforators, in contrast, are usually smaller in caliber and travel obliquely toward the lateral flank. They rarely cross the midline, instead mainly perfusing tissue on the *ipsilateral side*. In a flap depending on a lateral-row perforator, the portion across the midline (traditional Zone II) may receive very little flow, whereas the ipsilateral lateral portion (Zone III) is better perfused. This explains clinical observations that when a lateral perforator is used, surgeons often find the far medial side of the opposite side (old Zone II) ischemic first, whereas the lateral ipsilateral (old Zone III)

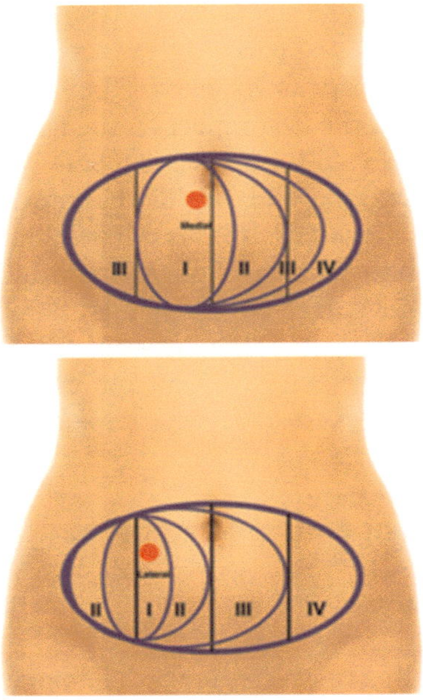

Figure 2.
Schematic diagram of perfusion zones (perforator angiosomes) in a lower abdominal flap, comparing a medialrow perforator (top) vs. a lateral-row perforator (bottom). The classic Hartrampf zones I–IV are marked for reference. A dominant medial perforator (red dot, top) supplies a broad central area and frequently perfuses across the midline (zone II), whereas the lateral extent (zone III) is somewhat less but still moderate. A dominant lateral perforator (red dot, bottom) primarily perfuses the ipsilateral side; its territory shifts laterally (making zone III relatively better perfused than zone II in this scenario). Zone IV (far contralateral) is least perfused in both cases. (This illustration is adapted from the model proposed by Rozen et al.).

can remain viable. **Figure 2** illustrates how the perfusion zones shift depending on a medial vs. lateral perforator.

The "Rozen's zones" or perforator angiosome model refines the classic four-zone concept by tailoring perfusion to the specific perforator used. A single perforator can reliably supply its own territory plus one adjacent "choke zone," but perfusion beyond this—such as reaching traditional Zone IV—usually exceeds anatomical limits unless true anastomoses exist, which are variable and unpredictable on current imaging. Medial-row perforators often supply larger, more central territories crossing the midline, while lateral-row perforators perfuse more lateralized areas. Modern planning with CTA allows surgeons to map these perforasomes, avoid poorly perfused distal tissue, and design flaps that respect vascular boundaries, thereby reducing fat necrosis and improving outcomes (**Figures 3** and **4**).

3.2 Pre-operative imaging

Modern perforator flap surgery relies on accurate pre-operative mapping of blood vessels to optimize flap design and minimize ischemic complications. Below, we discuss various imaging modalities and review the perfusion anatomy of the abdominal flap.

3.3 Doppler ultrasonography (handheld and duplex)

Doppler ultrasound has been a traditional, noninvasive tool for locating perforators. Early approaches used a simple handheld Doppler (HHD) probe to audibly detect

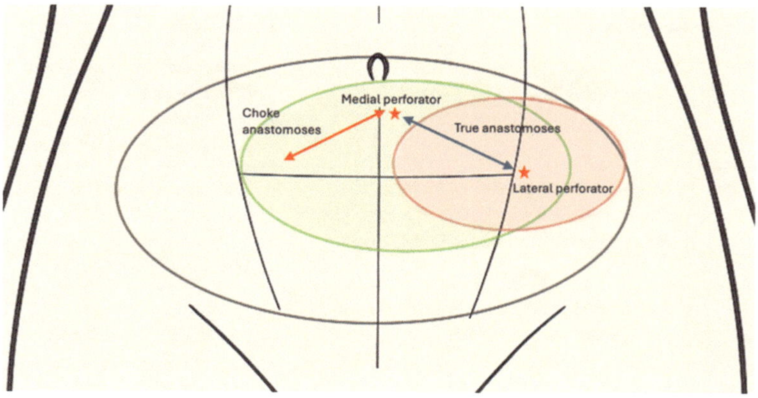

Figure 3.
Saint-Cyr's dynamic angiosome model showing overlapping perforator angiosomes (medial vs. lateral perforators) with direct (blue arrow) and choke (red arrow) vessel connections. Zones farther than one choke anastomosis from the source perforator have markedly diminished perfusion.

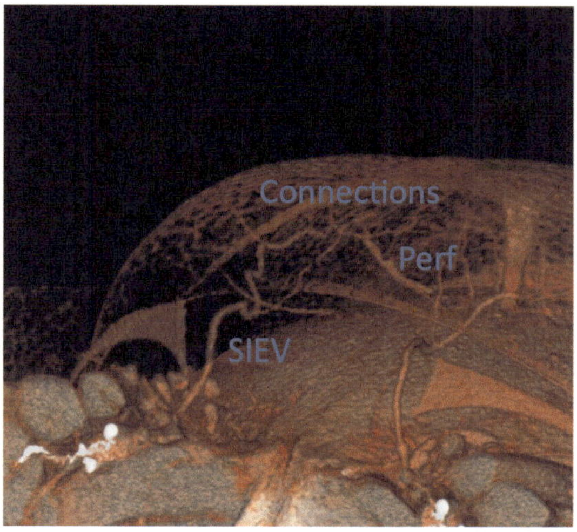

Figure 4.
3D volume rendering technique (VRT) image demonstrating the venous connections between the superficial inferior epigastric vein (SIEV) and the deep inferior epigastric artery (DIEA) perforators. The presence of robust interconnections supports adequate venous outflow through the deep system. In cases where such connections are absent or inadequate, prophylactic venous supercharging via *SIEV anastomosis is warranted to reduce the risk of postoperative venous congestion.*

the arterial signals on the skin. This method is quick, inexpensive, and involves no radiation or contrast, making it widely accessible. However, HHD provides no depth or course information and can produce false signals from non-target vessels (e.g., veins or small branches). Its specificity is limited—for example, studies have found that Doppler ultrasound had the lowest agreement with intraoperative findings (~74% concordance) among mapping methods [15].

Color duplex ultrasonography (CDUS) is a more advanced Doppler technique that visualizes the vessel while measuring blood flow. CDUS allows the estimation of perforator caliber and flow velocity and can differentiate artery vs. vein [16]. In experienced hands, ultrasound mapping can effectively identify dominant perforators —a 2023 randomized trial even found that surgeon-performed CDUS was not inferior

Modality	Advantages	Disadvantages
Handheld Doppler	• Simple, quick, widely available • No radiation or contrast needed	• Low specificity; may detect non-target vessels • No depth/course info (auditory only) • Operator-dependent interpretation
Color Duplex US	• Visualizes both arterial and venous flow (can measure diameter and velocity) [18] • No radiation; portable for bedside use	• Time-consuming and highly operator-dependent [19] • Provides anatomy but not extensive 3D course like CTA
CTA (CT Angiography)	• Excellent spatial resolution; detects perforators ~0.3 mm [20] • Shows intramuscular course, branches, and 3D anatomy • High sensitivity (~95–100%) • Reduces operative time and complications by guiding perforator choice [21]	• Exposure to radiation and IV contrast (small allergy/nephropathy risk) • Higher cost; requires radiologist and equipment • Static image (no real-time perfusion or flow info)
DIRT (Thermal imaging)	• Noninvasive, no contrast needed; low cost • Dynamically maps *functional* perfusion (hotspot rewarming indicates flow)	• Lower spatial resolution and no depth info • Susceptible to ambient conditions and patient factors • Limited evidence; typically an adjunct to other mapping methods
ICG fluorescence	• Real-time visualization of flap perfusion intraoperatively • Identifies ischemic areas for resection, improving safety • Repeatable (short dye half-life) [22]	• Intraoperative use only (no pre-op planning capability) • Requires specialized camera system and ICG dye • Additional cost per use (equipment and disposables)

Table 1.
Comparison of preoperative flap planning modalities (Doppler vs. CTA vs. advanced techniques).

to CTA for localizing DIEP perforators [17]. Despite these advantages, Doppler ultrasonography has important limitations. Results are highly operator-dependent and training/experience significantly impact accuracy [16]. **Table 1** compares Doppler with other modalities in perforator mapping.

3.4 Computed tomography angiography (CTA)

CTA has emerged as the gold standard for pre-operative perforator mapping in abdominal flaps [16]. High-resolution CTA can reliably detect perforators as small as ~0.3 mm [23], far better sensitivity than most other imaging modalities. It provides a precise map of perforator anatomy, including the location of each perforator relative to landmarks, its diameter, and its intramuscular trajectory through the rectus abdominis muscle. Further, it tells about perforator arborization, giving additional information about flap perfusion. Perforators can be categorized by row (medial vs. lateral) on the CTA, and their branching pattern in the subcutaneous fat can be visualized on reconstructed images (**Figure 5**). This rich anatomical detail allows surgeons to select the ideal perforator (e.g., largest caliber with short intramuscular course) and mark its location on the skin pre-operatively.

CTA planning has been linked to lower complication rates—including reduced partial flap necrosis and fat necrosis—compared to using handheld Doppler alone.

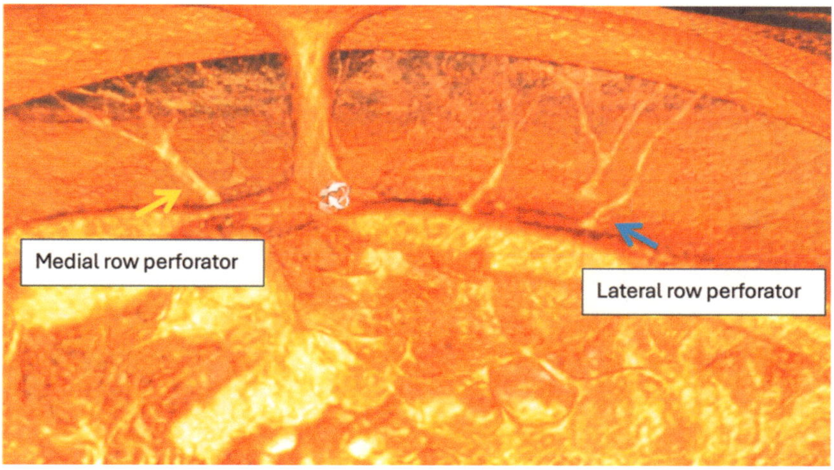

Figure 5.
Cranial view of 3D reconstruction showing clear separation between medial (yellow arrow) and lateral row (blue arrow) perforators at the level sectioned 4 cm above the umbilicus.

One cohort found that incorporating CTA cut operative costs by an average of $3000 per patient due to efficiency gains [23].

Despite its strengths, CTA has several disadvantages to consider. It exposes the patient to ionizing radiation and requires iodinated contrast injection, which carries a small risk of allergic reactions or contrast-induced nephropathy. (Modern low-osmolality contrast has allergy rates <1% and nephrotoxicity risk is low in patients without severe renal impairment.) Another limitation is that CTA provides a static anatomical snapshot—it shows the vessels but not the dynamic perfusion of the flap tissue. For instance, CTA cannot definitively tell how much skin territory a given perforator will supply (the "perforasome"), or whether choke vessels will carry blood to adjacent zones—it can only infer potential by showing vessel connections [24]. In practice, CTA's high sensitivity (approaching 95–100% for perforator detection) makes it an excellent map, but real-time perfusion assessment may still require other techniques intraoperatively. The skin markings are performed based on the perforators identified on CTA and marked on the skin surface (**Figure 6**).

3.5 Advanced flap design tools: Thermal imaging, 3D virtual reality, and ICG

In addition to Doppler and CTA, newer technologies are enhancing flap design by assessing perforator perfusion in innovative ways:

- *Dynamic infrared thermography (DIRT):* This technique uses a thermal camera to visualize skin temperature changes over time. After a region of skin is cooled (e.g., with an alcohol spray and fan), perforated skin areas will re-warm faster due to blood flow. On a thermographic map, active perforators appear as "hot spots" as the tissue heats back up. DIRT is noninvasive, painless, and low-cost, providing a dynamic picture of cutaneous blood supply [25]. However, DIRT has limited spatial resolution and depth: It localizes skin perfusion qualitatively but does not delineate the exact vessel path. It is best used as an adjunct to other mapping methods [26].

- *3D virtual reality (VR) imaging:* Virtual reality reconstructions take CTA data and create an immersive 3D model of the patient's abdominal vasculature. Using VR

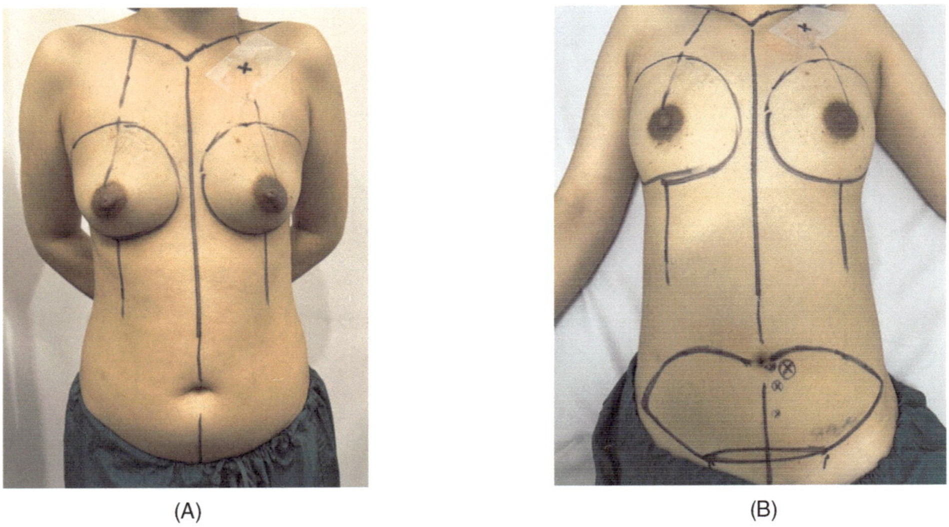

Figure 6.
(A) Preoperative skin markings performed in the standing position, showing the breast footprint, midline, breast meridian, and planned mastectomy incisions. This orientation accounts for natural breast position and symmetry. (B) Additional markings completed in the supine position, including the DIEP flap design and precise perforator locations as identified on preoperative CTA, ensuring the accurate alignment for flap harvest and inset.

headsets or 3D software, surgeons can "fly through" the abdominal wall and view perforators from any angle. A recent study compared traditional 2D CTA planning with a stereoscopic 3D-VR system: The VR model provided significantly more intuitive understanding of the perforators' course and branches, improving surgeons' confidence and speed in selecting perforators [27]. The VR visualization makes the intramuscular course and points of branching in the subcutaneous fat readily apparent in a single view, which can aid in deciding flap design (such as where to center the skin island). Some systems also integrate augmented reality (AR), allowing the projected perforator location to be overlaid on the patient's body for precise skin marking [27]. The main advantage of 3D VR is a better spatial understanding of complex anatomy, potentially leading to more accurate perforator selection in less time. Limitations include the need for specialized equipment/software and training to use it. VR is a new tool that uses existing CTA data to help surgeons interpret information more effectively.

- *Indocyanine green (ICG) fluorescence angiography:* ICG angiography is an intraoperative imaging technique to assess flap perfusion in real time. A near-infrared camera system (e.g., SPY) is used after intravenous injection of indocyanine green dye. ICG is very useful for confirming the perfusion of the flap and identifying any poorly perfused zones [24]. This helps reduce postoperative fat necrosis by allowing on-table adjustments. ICG angiography can also visualize choke vessel fill-over between perforator territories, indicating if adjacent angiosomes are being perfused through connecting vessels. The dye's short half-life permits multiple repeat evaluations in the same surgery if needed. It has minimal impact on operative time (each imaging run takes only a few minutes). The downsides are the requirement of specialized equipment and consumables (dye kits), as well as the fact it cannot be used pre-operatively—it is purely an intraoperative assessment tool. **Table 1** below offers a summary comparison of the above imaging and planning modalities:

4. Operative technique and workflow

4.1 Two-team surgical approach

A *two-team approach* is commonly employed to streamline DIEP flap breast reconstruction. One team (primary surgeon and assistant) focuses on harvesting the abdominal flap, while a second team concurrently prepares the chest recipient vessels [22]. Typically, the internal mammary artery and vein (IMA/IMV) or thoracodorsal artery and vein (TDA/TDV) are exposed as the recipient vessels of choice [28]. Using the internal mammary vessels facilitates optimal flap positioning (providing good medial breast fullness and symmetry) and requires a shorter pedicle length than using the axillary vessels [29]. In contrast, the thoracodorsal vessels are particularly advantageous in patients undergoing axillary clearance, as they are readily accessible within the same operative field, saving operative time and avoiding the need for rib resection.

4.2 Targeted perforator dissection ("running, walking, crawling")

Flap harvest in DIEP reconstruction progresses through three key dissection phases: suprafascial, intramuscular, and submuscular. The suprafascial or "running" phase involves rapid elevation of tissue above the rectus fascia to identify and clip minor perforators, focusing on the dominant one. Dissection here is broad and swift, as the risk of vascular injury is minimal. The intramuscular or "walking" phase begins once the fascia is incised around the chosen perforator, which is then carefully followed through the rectus muscle. This stage demands meticulous technique—using bipolar cautery and fine scissors—to preserve the fragile vessel and manage small branches. Finally, the submuscular or "crawling" phase entails delicate mobilization of the deep inferior epigastric artery and veins from beneath the muscle. This step provides maximal pedicle length but is technically demanding, requiring adequate retraction to avoid injury to the main vascular supply [4, 5].

Not all perforators take the same intramuscular course. Some favorable perforators have a paramuscular trajectory, meaning they run along the edge of the muscle or through natural septal planes rather than tunneling deep within the muscle fibers [30]. In about 10–15% of patients, a dominant perforator may emerge near the medial border of the rectus (paramuscular) and go to the skin without much muscle penetration. Dissecting such a perforator is generally easier and faster because minimal muscle fiber needs to be split—this reduces donor-site morbidity and risk of denervation to the muscle. However, gaining adequate pedicle length can be difficult. Often the surgeon must make a longer fascial incision to reach under the muscle and follow the DIEA pedicle back to its origin [30]. This can be technically demanding in a deep cavity and may require additional retraction. In other words, a paramuscular perforator spares muscle fiber cutting, but the submuscular pedicle dissection might be just as painstaking (or more so) to ensure the main artery and veins are safely freed.

4.3 Managing small perforators and conversion to MS-TRAM

A fundamental goal in DIEP surgery is to base the flap on an adequate perforator (or a small group of perforators) that can perfuse the entire skin-fat paddle. If only very small-caliber perforators are present, the surgeon faces a higher difficulty in dissection and a risk that perfusion may be marginal. Small perforators are also more

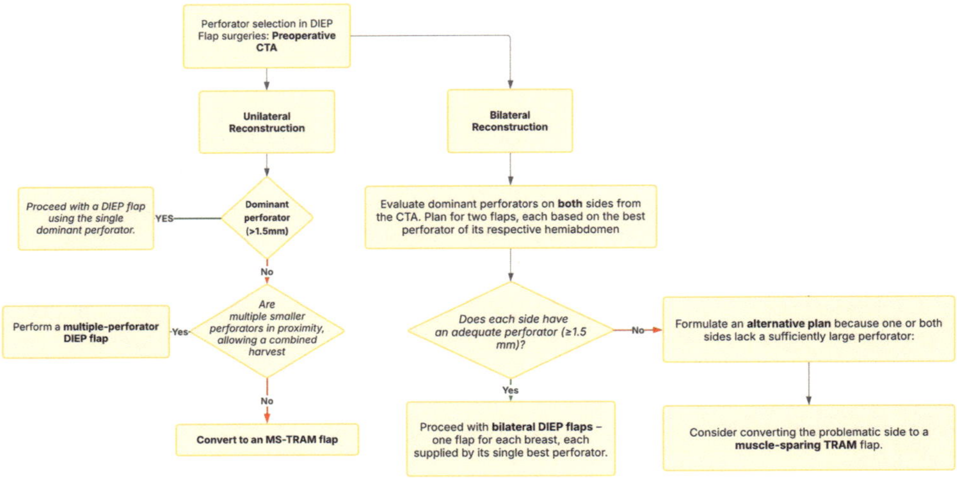

Figure 7.
Algorithm for perforator selection in DIEP flap surgery, illustrating decision pathways for unilateral vs. bilateral flaps and highlighting scenarios where multiple perforators or a muscle-sparing (MS) TRAM conversion may be utilized. Preoperative CTA imaging can guide the initial choice, but intraoperative findings might prompt switching to an MS-TRAM to ensure the flap's viability.

fragile, increasing the chance of intraoperative injury. To mitigate these issues, surgeons have a few strategies:

Intraoperative adjustments during DIEP flap harvest are sometimes necessary to ensure optimal perfusion. When multiple small perforators are found in close proximity—typically within the same intramuscular septum or along a single row—they can be harvested together through one muscle opening to enhance blood flow without compromising the muscle-sparing approach. In larger flaps or when a single perforator's flow is questionable, a "flow-through" or bipedicled approach may be employed, using two pedicles (e.g., bilateral DIEAs) and anastomosing each to separate recipient vessels. Alternatively, two perforators from the same side may be used in a Y-configuration to a single recipient artery. The presence of small perforators is a key indication for conversion from a pure DIEP flap to a muscle-sparing TRAM (MS-TRAM) flap. Additional indications include inadvertent intraoperative injury to one or more perforators, evidence of inadequate perfusion on intraoperative assessment, or previous abdominal surgery, where inclusion of a small segment of muscle with the vascular pedicle may be necessary to ensure more reliable vascularity [31, 32]. **Figure 7** depicts an algorithm for perforator selection in DIEP flap surgery, combining preoperative CTA guidance with intraoperative assessment to determine the optimal perforator(s) and the potential need for MS-TRAM conversion.

4.4 Recipient vessel preparation: Internal mammary vessels

The internal mammary vessels (typically the artery and vein in the 2nd or 3rd intercostal space) are the preferred recipients for DIEP flaps. Through the mastectomy incision, the surgeon identifies the intercostal space and carefully separates the costal cartilage to expose the internal mammary artery and vein. A rib-sparing technique may be used: Instead of removing an entire rib segment, often only a portion of cartilage is excised or the space is dilated to access the vessels [33]. This preserves chest wall integrity and reduces postoperative pain and contour deformities compared to older

DOI: http://dx.doi.org/10.5772/intechopen.1015108

rib-sacrificing methods [34]. Typically, the internal mammary vessels yield excellent inflow and outflow—the arterial pressure from the subclavian system and the "Venturi effect" of the large central veins help drive perfusion through the flap [35].

5. Venous supercharging

In abdominal free flaps (like DIEP or TRAM flaps), venous drainage occurs through the deep inferior epigastric veins (deep system) and the superficial inferior epigastric vein (SIEV, superficial system). Incorporating both systems *via* a second venous anastomosis can significantly improve venous drainage and prevent congestion [36]. Venous congestion is a major cause of flap complications (leading to partial flap loss or fat necrosis), especially in large flaps.

5.1 Options for venous supercharging

Several techniques and vein choices exist to supercharge venous outflow in autologous breast reconstruction flaps:

- *Use of the superficial inferior epigastric vein (SIEV):* The SIEV is preserved and anastomosed to a second recipient vein. A common approach is to anastomose the SIEV into the internal mammary vein system (e.g., to the second intercostal perforator or the retrograde limb of the internal mammary vein) [37, 38]. Studies report that performing an SIEV anastomosis to an internal mammary branch significantly reduces venous congestion and flap complications without adding substantial operative time. In one series, when a second vein (usually the SIEV) was used in DIEP flaps, venous congestion cases dropped to *zero* (0% vs. 2.6% in single-vein cases, $p = 0.006$). **Figure 8** depicts the setup for venous supercharging.

- *Alternate recipient veins:* Other options include the thoracodorsal or lateral thoracic vein in the axilla, or intercostal vein branches. For instance, the thoracodorsal system was used in ~62% of double-pedicle cases in one report and intercostal perforator veins in ~26%. The key is to choose a recipient that allows a tension-free anastomosis and good flow [39].

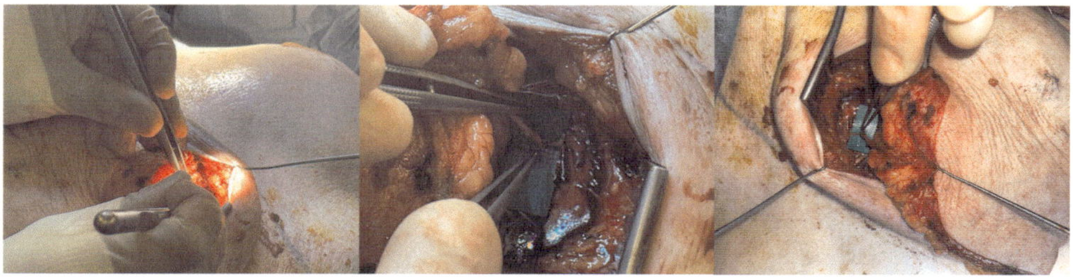

Figure 8.
Intraoperative view of venous supercharging during DIEP flap breast reconstruction. Additional retraction with skin hooks provides optimal exposure of the recipient site. The superficial inferior epigastric vein (SIEV) is seen being anastomosed end-to-end to the internal mammary perforator vein, establishing an auxiliary venous outflow pathway to reduce the risk of postoperative congestion.

- *Flow-through or retrograde techniques:* Another strategy is using the retrograde limb of the internal mammary vein when the main (antegrade) limb is occupied by the primary venous anastomosis [37]. A study using this dual-IMV approach reported *zero* cases of venous congestion or flap loss when two venous anastomoses were performed, versus some complications in single-vein cases.

- *Venous cross-over bypass:* Venous cross-over bypass using an interposition vein graft is a useful option when ipsilateral recipient veins are inadequate. In this technique, the flap vein—typically the SIEV or a vena comitans—is anastomosed to a vein graft and tunneled through a presternal subcutaneous plane to the contralateral internal mammary vein, providing an alternative route for venous drainage. Cannula venesection may also be used as a temporizing measure, involving cannulation of the SIEV to allow the controlled external drainage and relieve venous congestion until definitive venous outflow is established.

- *Prophylactic supercharging to prevent fat necrosis:* Rather than waiting for signs of venous compromise, many surgeons now advocate routine (prophylactic) venous supercharging in large or high-risk flaps to preempt problems. Evidence is mounting that this practice can reduce complications like fat necrosis. A 2024 study showed that routine SIEV augmentation in DIEP flaps significantly lowered the combined risk of venous complications and fat necrosis (hazard ratio $\sim$ 0.33, $p = 0.0489$). Importantly, this benefit was observed regardless of flap weight (even though supercharged flaps tended to be heavier on average) [38]. Similarly, a meta-analysis of multiple studies confirmed a *statistically significant* reduction in partial flap necrosis (RR $\sim$0.50) and total flap loss (RR $\sim$0.31) when a second vein was used. In practical terms, flaps with dual venous drainage had markedly lower rates of fat necrosis compared to single-vein flaps [40]. No appreciable increase in operative time or morbidity was noted with adding a venous anastomosis, making prophylactic supercharging a safe preventive measure.

6. Handling surgical challenges and complex cases

Certain patient situations and anatomical challenges can complicate flap-based breast reconstruction. Below we discuss how to handle complex cases, including previously operated abdomens (scars, hernias), stacked or bipedicled flap techniques for added volume, prior liposuction to the donor site, and large chest wall defects.

6.1 Previously operated abdomen (scars and hernias)

In the past, prior abdominal surgery was often viewed as a relative contraindication to using abdominal flaps [41]. However, modern experience shows that most abdominal scars do not preclude successful DIEP/MS-TRAM flap harvest, provided careful planning is done. Preoperative imaging (CT or MR angiography) is extremely helpful—it can map out the perforators and their course around scars. For routine scars like appendectomy, laparoscopic ports, or C-sections, surgeons typically adjust the flap layout to ensure key perforators are included in the flap away from the scar tissue. Large midline scars (from prior open surgeries) may require the surgeon to use tissue from one side of the abdomen or even consider a bipedicled flap (using both sides) to ensure perfusion across the midline. In challenging cases (e.g., multiple

DOI: http://dx.doi.org/10.5772/intechopen.1015108

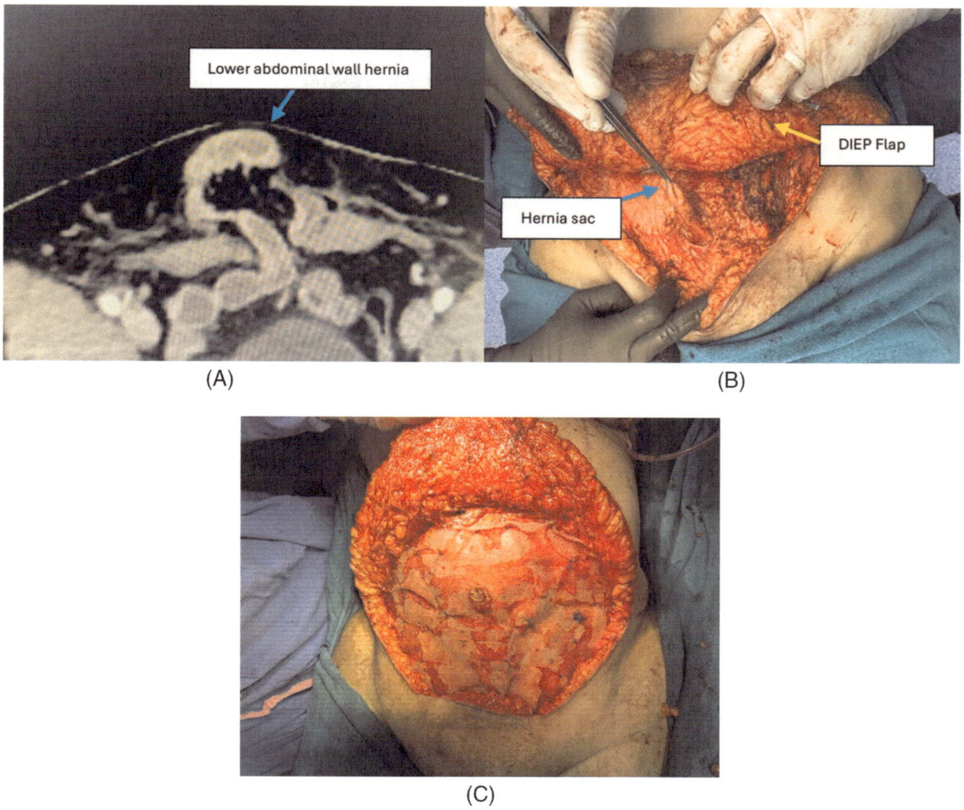

Figure 9.
DIEP flap harvest in a patient with a lower midline cesarean scar hernia. (A) Axial CTA image showing a midline fascial defect consistent with an incisional hernia, with herniated bowel loops. (B) Intraoperative view demonstrating the hernia sac held with forceps, adjacent to the raised DIEP flap being elevated by the surgeon. Despite the presence of a midline hernia, the flap was successfully harvested with careful dissection and preservation of perforators. (C) The anterior abdominal was strengthened using a 30x30-cm prolene mesh as shown.

abdominal surgeries), alternatives like a PAP or latissimus flap can be backups, but abdominal flaps often remain feasible with ingenuity.

If a ventral hernia or mesh is present, additional care is needed. A small, easily reducible hernia can be repaired at the time of flap harvest (sometimes the flap harvest itself incorporates hernia repair by tightening the abdominal wall). The presence of synthetic mesh from a prior hernia repair can make dissection more difficult due to scarring; it may also indicate some perforators are damaged or encased in scar. Surgeons can sometimes work around or even remove a portion of mesh if it lies in the flap territory. Every case is unique—minor hernias generally do not prevent a DIEP flap, whereas a history of abdominoplasty (tummy tuck) is a contraindication because the central perforators have been cut out with the excess skin resection (**Figure 9**).

6.2 Stacked and bipedicled flaps for increased volume

Some patients require more tissue than a single abdominal flap can provide. In such cases, innovative techniques like *stacked* or *bipedicled* flaps are employed to achieve the desired volume:

- *Stacked flaps:* A stacked flap procedure involves transferring two free flaps and layering them ("stacking") to create one breast mound. In practice, this often means both sides of the lower abdomen are harvested as separate DIEP flaps—one for the upper pole and one for the lower pole of the breast—and transplanted to the same breast. Each flap has its own pedicle and is anastomosed to recipient vessels (sometimes to a single recipient artery with a Y-connection, or to separate recipient sites) [42].

- *Bipedicled flaps:* A bipedicled abdominal flap uses two pedicles for one large flap, effectively treating the entire abdominal pannus as one unit. The surgeon harvests the entire lower abdomen skin-fat as one piece but includes perforators (and DIEA vessels) from both sides. This yields a *42+ cm wide flap* in some cases [43]. Each side's pedicle is then anastomosed to recipient vessels—for example, the right DIEP vessels to the right internal mammary, and the left DIEP vessels to the left internal mammary (or to thoracodorsal vessels). The result is a single massive flap with dual blood supply. Bipedicled DIEP flaps (also called double-pedicle flaps) are especially useful in large bilateral chest defects or for very large unilateral reconstructions. They allow all four zones of the abdominal tissue to be used in one breast reconstruction, maximizing volume.

Both stacked and bipedicled techniques enable the surgeon to overcome volume limitations of a single flap. They are resource-intensive (two donor sites or two pedicles), but for the right indication—such as a patient with a small abdomen and large chest requirement—they provide an autologous solution when one flap would not suffice [44].

6.3 Chest wall resurfacing and other complex situations

In some breast cancer or oncologic cases, the challenge is not just volume replacement but also coverage of a large chest wall defect. For instance, a locally advanced

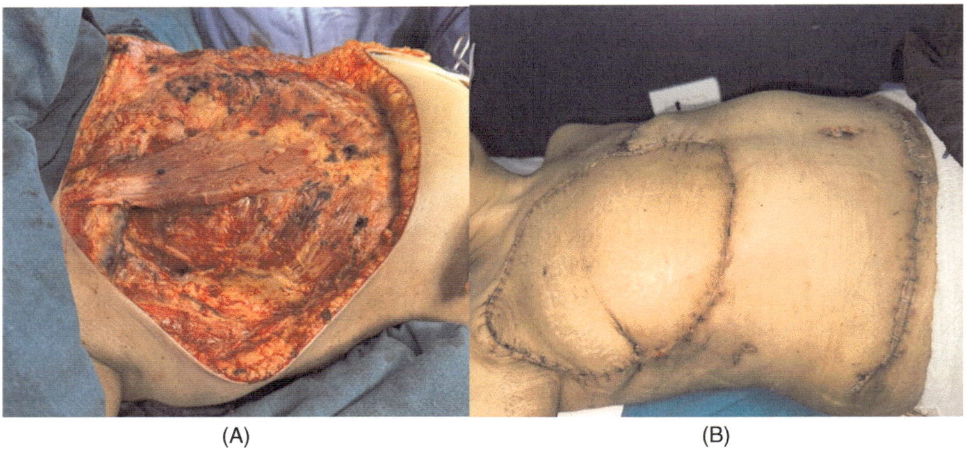

Figure 10.
Bipedicled DIEP flap for massive chest wall reconstruction. (A) Extensive anterior chest wall defect following radical mastectomy. (B) Well-settled bipedicled DIEP flap providing durable, well-vascularized soft tissue coverage.

tumor resection might remove significant chest skin, muscle (pectoralis), or even parts of the chest wall, leaving a massive wound. A bipedicled DIEP flap for chest wall reconstruction has been reported as a promising solution for extensive anterior chest defects [45]. Using the full abdominal skin island, a bipedicled flap can span from clavicle to mid-abdomen, covering a broad area with well-vascularized tissue. This approach provides robust soft-tissue coverage to protect underlying structures (ribs, implants, etc.) while still sparing the abdominal muscles (since it is perforator-based). Other flaps like the latissimus dorsi or omental flaps have roles in chest wall reconstruction, but abdominal perforator flaps offer the advantage of bringing in a large skin paddle and ample tissue in one transfer (**Figure 10**).

7. The future of breast reconstruction

The future of breast reconstruction is poised for transformative change through integration of emerging surgical and imaging technologies. Robotic-assisted harvests, particularly with systems like the da Vinci and dedicated microsurgical robots such as Symani®, promise enhanced precision, tremor elimination, and access to deep or narrow anatomical spaces with minimal trauma [46]. Robotic microsurgery is already demonstrating feasibility for supermicrosurgical anastomoses in lymphatic and perforator surgery, and its application to DIEP flap dissection and vessel coupling may shorten learning curves and improve consistency [46, 47]. Advances in perfusion assessment—such as real-time hyperspectral imaging, including Laser Speckle Contrast Imaging (LSCI) for measuring tissue oxygenation and perfusion, and quantitative analysis software (SPY-Q)—enable objective and quantitative analysis of flap perfusion. AI-enhanced indocyanine green angiography (ICG-A), such as the SPY Elite system, further helps identify the perfusion gradients and provides quantitative, continuous monitoring of flap vascularity, thereby enabling more precise and dynamic intraoperative decision-making.

8. Conclusion

DIEP flap breast reconstruction is the gold standard for autologous reconstruction, offering excellent esthetic outcomes with minimal donor site morbidity. Consistent success relies on a structured, imaging-guided workflow, including preoperative CT angiography for precise perforator selection, meticulous perforator dissection, and adjunctive techniques such as venous supercharging to optimize perfusion and reduce complications. A standardized two-team approach enhances operative efficiency, facilitates training, and improves reproducibility. The integration of emerging advanced perfusion assessment and imaging technologies into clinical protocols is expected to provide the immediate, actionable intraoperative data, further improving surgical precision and overall success rates in breast reconstruction.

Acknowledgements

The author acknowledges the use of Chat GPT for language polishing of the manuscript.

Conflict of interest

The authors declare no conflict of interest.

Abbreviations

DIEP	deep inferior epigastric perforator
TRAM	transverse rectus abdominis myocutaneous
CTA	computed tomographic angiography
DIRT	dynamic infrared thermography
ICG	indocyanine green
SIEV	superficial inferior epigastric vein
DIEA	deep inferior epigastric artery
IMA/IMV	internal mammary artery/internal mammary vein
PAP flap	profunda artery perforator flap
VR	virtual reality
AR	augmented reality
MS-TRAM	muscle-sparing transverse rectus abdominis myocutaneous flap

Author details

Samarth Gupta[1]* and Venkat Ramakrishnan[2]

1 Apollo Athenaa Women's Cancer Centre, Delhi, India

2 St. Andrew's Centre for Plastic Surgery, Chelmsford, UK

*Address all correspondence to: guptasamarth@hotmail.com

References

[1] Nahabedian M, Schwartz J. Autologous breast reconstruction following mastectomy. Handchirurgie Mikrochirurgie Plastische Chirurgie. 2008;**40**(04):248-254. DOI: 10.1055/s-2008-1038754

[2] Nahabedian MY. The deep inferior epigastric perforator flap: Where we started and where we are now. Gland Surgery. 2023;**12**(5):696-703. DOI: 10.21037/gs-22-636

[3] Allen RJ, Treece P. Deep inferior epigastric perforator flap for breast reconstruction. Annals of Plastic Surgery. 1994;**32**(1):32-38. DOI: 10.1097/00000637-199401000-00007

[4] Haddock NT, Kayfan S, Pezeshk RA, Teotia SS. Co-surgeons in breast reconstructive microsurgery: What do they bring to the table? Microsurgery. 2018;**38**(1):14-20. DOI: 10.1002/micr.30191

[5] Withers J et al. 69. Combating the learning curve for DIEP flaps: Preliminary results from a cognitive task analysis study. Plastic and Reconstructive Surgery. Global Open. 2024;**12**(S4):47-48. DOI: 10.1097/01.GOX.0001015368.72135.9d

[6] Holmström H. The free abdominoplasty flap and its use in breast reconstruction. An experimental study and clinical case report. Scandinavian Journal of Plastic and Reconstructive Surgery. 1979;**13**(3):423-427. DOI: 10.3109/02844317909013092

[7] Hartrampf CR, Scheflan M, Black PW. Breast reconstruction with a transverse abdominal Island flap. Plastic and Reconstructive Surgery. 1982;**69**(2):216-224. DOI: 10.1097/00006534-198202000-00006

[8] Blondeel PN, Boeckx WD. Refinements in free flap breast reconstruction: The free bilateral deep inferior epigastric perforator flap anastomosed to the internal mammary artery. British Journal of Plastic Surgery. 1994;**47**(7):495-501. DOI: 10.1016/0007-1226(94)90033-7

[9] Arya R, Healy C, Frame JD, Ramakrishnan V. 21 year follow up of a DIEP (deep inferior epigastric perforator) flap: A tale of a 'nulltiple,'. Journal of Plastic, Reconstructive & Aesthetic Surgery. 2014;**67**(10):1436-1439. DOI: 10.1016/j.bjps.2014.04.028

[10] Blondeel PN. One hundred free DIEP flap breast reconstructions: A personal experience. British Journal of Plastic Surgery. 1999;**52**(2):104-111. DOI: 10.1054/bjps.1998.3033

[11] Connon FV, Taylor GI, Gascoigne AC, Corlett RJ, Ashton MW. Understanding the vascular anatomy of zone IV in DIEA perforator flaps. Australasian Journal of Plastic Surgery. 2018;**1**(1):86-95. DOI: 10.34239/ajops.v1i1.38

[12] Dinner MI, Dowden RV, Scheflan M. Refinements in the use of the transverse abdominal Island flap for postmastectomy reconstruction. Annals of Plastic Surgery. 1983;**11**(5):362-372. DOI: 10.1097/00000637-198311000-00002

[13] Saint-Cyr M. Assessing perforator architecture. Clinics in Plastic Surgery. 2011;**38**(2):175-202. DOI: 10.1016/j.cps.2011.03.015

[14] Rozen WM, Ashton MW, Le Roux CM, Pan W, Corlett RJ. The perforator angiosome: A new concept in

the design of deep inferior epigastric artery perforator flaps for breast reconstruction. Microsurgery. 2010;**30**(1):1-7. DOI: 10.1002/micr.20684

[15] Kiely J, Kumar M, Wade RG. The accuracy of different modalities of perforator mapping for unilateral DIEP flap breast reconstruction: A systematic review and meta-analysis. Journal of Plastic, Reconstructive & Aesthetic Surgery. 2021;**74**(5):945-956. DOI: 10.1016/j.bjps.2020.12.005

[16] Orădan AV et al. The precision of colour Doppler ultrasonography combined with dynamic infrared thermography in perforator mapping for deep inferior epigastric perforator flap breast reconstruction. Journal of Personalized Medicine. 2024;**14**(9):969. DOI: 10.3390/jpm14090969

[17] Bajus A et al. Color Doppler ultrasound versus CT angiography for DIEP flap planning: A randomized controlled trial. Journal of Plastic, Reconstructive & Aesthetic Surgery. 2023;**86**:48-57. DOI: 10.1016/j.bjps.2023.07.042

[18] Lovětínská V et al. Stable arterial perforators mapping in lower leg using color-coded Doppler sonography, acoustic Doppler, and thermal imaging camera in patients undergoing digital subtraction angiography. Journal of Reconstructive Microsurgery Open. 2024;**09**(01):e52-e63. DOI: 10.1055/a-2241-2323

[19] Steenbeek LM, Peperkamp K, Ulrich DJO, Hummelink S. Alternative imaging technologies for perforator mapping in free flap breast reconstructive surgery – A comprehensive overview of the current literature. Journal of Plastic, Reconstructive & Aesthetic Surgery. 2022;**75**(11):4074-4084. DOI: 10.1016/j.bjps.2022.06.100

[20] Rozen W, Ashton M, Stella D, Phillips TJ, Taylor G. Magnetic resonance angiography and computed tomographic angiography for free fibular flap transfer. Journal of Reconstructive Microsurgery. 2008;**24**(06):457-458. DOI: 10.1055/s-0028-1082890

[21] Thiessen FEF et al. Dynamic infrared thermography (DIRT) in DIEP flap breast reconstruction: A clinical study with a standardized measurement setup. European Journal of Obstetrics & Gynecology and Reproductive Biology. 2020;**252**:166-173. DOI: 10.1016/j.ejogrb.2020.05.038

[22] Andreas W, Jones GE, editor. 53 DIEP flap reconstruction and technique. In: Bostwick's Plastic and Reconstructive Breast Surgery. Stuttgart: Georg Thieme Verlag; 2020. DOI: 10.1055/b-0040-176819

[23] Nassar AH et al. Comparison of various modalities utilized for preoperative planning in microsurgical reconstructive surgery. Journal of Reconstructive Microsurgery. 2022; **38**(03):170-180. DOI: 10.1055/s-0041-1736316

[24] Rozen WM, Leung R, Chae MP, Hunter-Smith DJ. Imaging of perforasome territories: The evolution of techniques. Australasian Journal of Plastic Surgery. 2018;**1**(2):52-60. DOI: 10.34239/ajops.v1i2.121

[25] Muntean MV. Using dynamic infrared thermography to optimize color Doppler ultrasound mapping of cutaneous perforators. Medical Ultrasonography. 2015;**17**(4):503-507. DOI: 10.11152/mu.2013.2066.174.dyn

[26] Sonda R et al. Deep inferior epigastric perforator flap preoperative

planning: A comparative analysis between dynamic infrared thermography, computerized tomography angiography, and hand-held Doppler. Microsurgery. 2022;**42**(7):649-658. DOI: 10.1002/micr.30927

[27] Di Via Ioschpe A, Golijanin B, Benharush D, Berl A, Perhulov V, Egozi D. Preoperative planning using virtual reality and computed tomography angiogram in deep inferior epigastric perforator flap breast reconstruction. Journal of Plastic, Reconstructive & Aesthetic Surgery. 2023;**87**:161-169. DOI: 10.1016/j.bjps.2023.08.004

[28] Rosich-Medina A, Bouloumpasis S, Di Candia M, Malata CM. Total 'rib'-preservation technique of internal mammary vessel exposure for free flap breast reconstruction: A 5-year prospective cohort study and instructional video. Annals of Medicine and Surgery (London). 2015;**4**(3):293-300. DOI: 10.1016/j.amsu.2015.08.006

[29] Arnež ZM, Valdatta L, Tyler MP, Planinšek F. Anatomy of the internal mammary veins and their use in free TRAM flap breast reconstruction. British Journal of Plastic Surgery. 1995;**48**(8):540-545. DOI: 10.1016/0007-1226(95)90041-1

[30] Pons G, Masia J, Sanchez-Porro L, Larrañaga J, Clavero JA. Paramuscular perforators in DIEAP flap for breast reconstruction. Annals of Plastic Surgery. 2014;**73**(6):659-661. DOI: 10.1097/SAP.0b013e318285873e

[31] Martinez CA, Fairchild B, Secchi-del Rio R, Boutros SG. Bilateral outpatient breast reconstruction with stacked DIEP and vertical PAP flaps. Plastic and Reconstructive Surgery. Global Open. 2021;**9**(10):e3878. DOI: 10.1097/GOX.0000000000003878

[32] DellaCroce FJ et al. Myth-busting the DIEP flap and an introduction to the abdominal perforator exchange (APEX) breast reconstruction technique: A single-surgeon retrospective review. Plastic and Reconstructive Surgery. 2019;**143**(4):992-1008. DOI: 10.1097/PRS.0000000000005484

[33] Nejedlý A, Tvrdek M, Kletenský J, Pros Z. Internal mammary vessels as recipient vessels to the free TRAM flap. Acta Chirurgiae Plasticae. 1995;**37**(1):17-19

[34] Dupin CL, Allen RJ, Glass CA, Bunch R. The internal mammary artery and vein as a recipient site for free-flap breast reconstruction: A report of 110 consecutive cases. Plastic and Reconstructive Surgery. 1996;**98**:685-689. DOI: 10.1097/00006534-199609001-00013

[35] Quaba O, Brown A, Stevenson H. Internal mammary vessels, recipient vessels of choice for free tissue breast reconstruction? British Journal of Plastic Surgery. 2005;**58**(6):881-882. DOI: 10.1016/j.bjps.2005.04.005

[36] Enajat M, Rozen WM, Whitaker IS, Smit JM, Acosta R. A single center comparison of one versus two venous anastomoses in 564 consecutive DIEP flaps: Investigating the effect on venous congestion and flap survival. Microsurgery. 2010;**30**(3):185-191. DOI: 10.1002/micr.20712

[37] Lombardo GAG et al. Prophylactic venous supercharging in deep inferior epigastric artery perforator flap surgery: A retrospective dual-center study. Journal of Reconstructive Microsurgery. 2025;**41**(04):295-301. DOI: 10.1055/a-2355-3875

[38] Germann A et al. The effect of venous augmentation on complication rates in deep inferior epigastric perforator breast reconstruction. Microsurgery. 2024;**44**(7):e31220. DOI: 10.1002/micr.31220

[39] Patel NG et al. Stacked and bipedicled abdominal free flaps for breast reconstruction: Considerations for shaping. Gland Surgery. 2016;**5**(2): 115-121. DOI: 10.3978/j.issn.2227-684X.2016.02.03

[40] Pignatti M et al. Meta-analysis of the effects of venous super-drainage in deep inferior epigastric artery perforator flaps for breast reconstruction. Microsurgery. 2021;**41**(2):186-195. DOI: 10.1002/micr.30682

[41] Salgarello M, Barone-Adesi L, Cina A, Farallo E. The effect of liposuction on inferior epigastric perforator vessels. Annals of Plastic Surgery. 2005;**55**(4):346-351. DOI: 10.1097/01.sap.0000179168.69667.43

[42] DellaCroce FJ, Sullivan SK, Trahan C. Stacked deep inferior epigastric perforator flap breast reconstruction: A review of 110 flaps in 55 cases over 3 years. Plastic and Reconstructive Surgery. 2011;**127**(3): 1093-1099. DOI: 10.1097/PRS.0b013e318205f223

[43] Gupta S, Arora R, Mishra KS, Kumar A, Prasad N. Reconstruction of massive Chest Wall defect after bilateral mastectomy using a Bipedicled deep inferior epigastric perforator flap: A case report. International Microsurgery Journal. 2025;**9**(1):3. DOI: 10.24983/scitemed.imj.2025.00198

[44] Rabey NG, Erel E, Malata CM. Double-Pedicled abdominal free flap using an entirely new microvascular combination of DIEP and SIEA vascular pedicles for unilateral breast reconstruction. Plastic and Reconstructive Surgery. 2012;**130**(5): 767e-769e. DOI: 10.1097/PRS.0b013e318267d995

[45] Jessop Z, Thongvitokomarn S, Maclean G, Roy PG. Chest wall perforator flaps for chest wall resurfacing following mastectomy for locally advanced or recurrent breast cancer – A systematic review of the literature and our experience. European Journal of Surgical Oncology. 2024;**50**: 108111. DOI: 10.1016/j.ejso.2024.108111

[46] Sørensen RBA, Chakari W, Thomsen JB, Sørensen JA. Evaluation of microsurgical free flap procedures utilizing the Symani surgical system: A preliminary analysis. Journal of Plastic, Reconstructive & Aesthetic Surgery. 2025;**102**:66-70. DOI: 10.1016/j.bjps.2025.01.037

[47] Daar DA et al. Robotic deep inferior epigastric perforator flap harvest in breast reconstruction. Microsurgery. 2022;**42**(4):319-325. DOI: 10.1002/micr.30856

Chapter 4

Tendon Surgery for Thigh Injury in Professional Football Players

Loris Perticarini, Luca Andriollo and Francesco Benazzo

Abstract

Thigh muscle-tendon injuries are among the most frequent and disabling conditions in elite football, often leading to significant time loss, reduced performance, and high recurrence rates. The hamstrings, adductors, and rectus femoris are the most affected muscle groups, each with specific anatomical and biomechanical features influencing prognosis and management. Although the majority of injuries can be successfully managed conservatively, severe tendon lesions such as proximal avulsions, intratendinous ruptures, or recurrent injuries frequently require surgical intervention. Advances in diagnostic imaging and standardized classification systems have improved lesion characterization and guided treatment strategies, but clinical decision-making still relies on careful integration of anatomical, functional, and sport-specific factors. Surgical repair, when indicated, can restore tendon continuity, reduce recurrence risk, and enable a timely return to play, especially in high-performance athletes. Postoperative rehabilitation protocols must be tailored to the injury site and severity, with progressive loading, eccentric training, and sport-specific drills. A comprehensive understanding of reinjury mechanisms and individualized management strategies is essential to optimize outcomes and preserve athletic careers.

Keywords: thigh tendon injuries, hamstrings, quadriceps, rectus femoris, adductor, reinjury, surgery, football, rehabilitation

1. Introduction

Thigh muscle-tendon injuries represent a significant challenge in elite football, both because of their high incidence and their potential impact on player availability, performance, and career longevity. Muscle-tendon lesions account for approximately one-third of all time lost due to injuries in professional male football, with the vast majority (92%) affecting the lower limb's major muscle groups [1–4]. Within the thigh, injuries are classically grouped into three anatomical compartments: the posterior (hamstrings), the medial (adductors), and the anterior (quadriceps, particularly the rectus femoris).

Hamstring injuries are the most common, representing around 37% of thigh muscle-tendon injuries, followed by adductor injuries (23%) and quadriceps or rectus femoris injuries (19%) [1, 2, 5]. Hamstring strain injuries are the most prevalent noncontact lesions in professional men's football, often sustained during high-speed running or rapid changes of direction [6–8]. Adductor longus injuries are the leading cause of acute groin pain in footballers and frequently occur during kicking or change-of-direction actions [9, 10]. Quadriceps and rectus femoris injuries, while less frequent, can still lead to prolonged absence, particularly when tendon involvement is present [11].

Although the majority of these injuries recover with nonoperative management, severe tendon ruptures or avulsions, especially in the proximal hamstring, adductor longus, or rectus femoris, may require surgical repair [1, 10]. Across all compartments, severe injuries that result in more than 28 days of absence account for approximately 11% of muscle-tendon lesions in elite football [1]. Recurrence rates remain high despite advances in prevention and rehabilitation [12, 13].

A clear understanding of compartment-specific anatomy, injury mechanisms, and sport-specific epidemiology is essential for tailoring both prevention and treatment strategies in professional football. From a surgical perspective, early recognition of lesions at risk for poor healing is critical. Complete tendon avulsions, high-grade partial tears with significant retraction, and injuries involving key tendinous structures often require prompt operative management. Timely surgical intervention in these selected cases can improve return-to-play (RTP) rates, restore function, and reduce the likelihood of chronic symptoms or career-limiting deficits.

2. Diagnosis and classification of muscle-tendon injuries

2.1 Diagnostic imaging

Early and accurate diagnosis of thigh muscle-tendon injuries is crucial for optimal management and prognosis. Ultrasound (US) and MRI remain the preferred modalities for confirming the diagnosis and assessing lesion characteristics [14].

US offers portability, cost-effectiveness, and the advantage of dynamic, real-time evaluation during muscle contraction or stretching. In the acute phase (<2 weeks), US demonstrates high sensitivity for detecting fiber disruption, hematoma, and avulsion injuries [15, 16]. It is particularly useful for monitoring healing progression during rehabilitation. However, sensitivity declines as acute fluid resolves, and small distal musculotendinous junction (MTJ) lesions or subtle intratendinous tears may be missed [17].

MRI provides superior visualization of deep MTJ injuries, tendon retraction, and avulsion morphology [18]. MRI maintains diagnostic accuracy beyond the acute phase and may help estimate RTP timelines based on lesion length, cross-sectional area, and tendon involvement [19]. Optimal image acquisition is typically within 24–72 hours after injury and ideally within 1–2 weeks if surgical intervention is being considered [18]. Nevertheless, MRI grading alone has limited reliability in predicting exact RTP readiness [20].

2.2 Classification systems

Classification systems integrate clinical and imaging findings to standardize diagnosis, guide prognosis, and plan rehabilitation. Despite several proposals, no system consistently predicts RTP with high accuracy [21].

- Traditional Clinical Grading (Grade I–III) categorizes injuries based on structural disruption and strength loss [22]. Although widely used, its prognostic value is limited and does not account for anatomical location or tissue type.

- BAMIC – British Athletics Muscle Injury Classification assigns grades 0–4 based on MRI and clinical data, while differentiating anatomical location (myofascial, MTJ, intratendinous) [14, 23]. This location-based approach is clinically relevant, as intratendinous injuries often require longer rehabilitation. BAMIC demonstrates high inter- and intra-rater reliability [24] and offers structured rehabilitation guidelines, with reasonable prognostic correlation to RTP and reinjury risk [23, 25].

- In **Table 1**, the BAMIC classification is reported.

- Munich Consensus Classification distinguishes between functional and structural injuries and incorporates both mechanism and imaging findings [26]. Although comprehensive, its predictive accuracy for RTP duration remains inconsistent [27].

The Italian Society of Muscles, Ligaments and Tendons (ISMuLT) muscle injury classification established a standardized international terminology to align clinicians, radiologists, and rehabilitation specialists [28, 29]. It emphasizes the integration of clinical assessment with imaging findings and discourages ambiguous terms such as "elongation" or "strain." Prognosis is influenced not only by lesion size but also by

Grade	Anatomical location	Combined classification
Grade 0 Negative MRI		0a: Normal MRI *0b*: Normal or patchy high signal changes throughout one or more muscles
Grade 1 Small injuries (tears) to the muscle	a Myofascial b Musculotendinous c Intratendon	1a: High signal changes evident at the fascial border 1b: High signal changes <10% MTJ; longitudinal length < 5 cm (fiber disruption <1 cm may be present) *1c*: High signal changes extend into the tendon with longitudinal involvement <1 cm
Grade 2 Moderate injuries (tears) to the muscle		2a: High signal changes at fascial border with extension into muscle; CSA 10–50% at maximal site; length > 5 cm 2b: High signal changes at MTJ; CSA 10–50% at maximal site; length > 5 cm *2c*: High signal changes extend into the tendon; longitudinal tendon involvement >5 cm
Grade 3 Extensive tears (to the muscle)		3a: High signal changes at fascial border with muscle extension; CSA >50% at maximal site; length > 15 cm; architectural fiber disruption usually >5 cm 3b: High signal changes CSA >50% at maximal site; length > 15 cm; fiber disruption usually >5 cm *3c*: High signal changes extend into the tendon; tendon involvement >5 cm; CSA of tendon involvement >50% (possible loss of tendon tension, no discontinuity evident)
Grade 4 Complete tears (to either muscle or tendon)		4b: Complete discontinuity of the muscle with retraction *4c*: Complete discontinuity of the tendon with retraction

CSA: Cross-sectional area; MTJ: Musculotendinous junction.

Table 1.
British athletics muscle injury classification.

muscle- and tissue-specific factors. Injuries differ in outcome depending on whether they are proximal, mid-belly, or distal, and on the structures involved (myofascial, musculotendinous, or intratendinous). Healing and recovery times, therefore, vary by location, and prognosis further differs between first-time and recurrent injuries.

Overall, systems like BAMIC and ISMuLT muscle injury classification have improved standardization and clinical utility, particularly in differentiating injury sites and tissue involvement, which is essential for rehabilitation planning. However, variability in subcategories and the multifactorial nature of recovery mean that clinical assessment remains indispensable alongside imaging-based classification.

3. Hamstring injuries

The anatomy and biomechanics of the hamstrings are reported in Appendix A.

3.1 Epidemiology and risk factors in professional football

Hamstring strain injuries are the most common noncontact muscle injuries in professional football, representing 17–26% of all football-related lesions and up to one-third of all muscle injuries in elite players [6–8]. Despite preventive efforts, their incidence continues to rise by approximately 2.3% annually in top-level football. The biceps femoris long head is the muscle most frequently affected [7].

In elite European football, the injury rate is around 1.2 per 1000 exposure hours, with match incidence up to nine times higher than during training [7]. Approximately 22% of players sustain at least one hamstring injury each season, and recurrence is common, affecting over 30% of athletes, most often within the first competitive season after the initial injury [30–32].

RTP time depends on lesion type: Functional injuries average 6 days of absence, structural injuries about 18 days, with intratendinous lesions requiring 2–4 months [33]. Proximal tendon injuries tend to have longer recovery times than distal or myofascial injuries.

The risk of hamstring injuries increases with age. Although youth players show a lower incidence, the time lost per injury is comparable to that of adults [24]. Factors such as high sprinting demands, frequent kicking, and competitive intensity significantly contribute to the persistent burden of hamstring injuries in professional football [8].

3.2 Clinical assessment

Early and accurate diagnosis of hamstring strain injuries is essential for guiding treatment and optimizing RTP outcomes. However, prognosis remains difficult to determine due to the wide variability in injury grade, anatomical location, and mechanism [22, 34]. In professional football, the high recurrence rate and the potential for underdiagnosed low-grade injuries further complicate clinical management [8].

In elite football, approximately two-thirds of acute hamstring strain injuries affect the biceps femoris, with the remainder involving the semitendinosus or semimembranosus; up to 30% involve multiple muscles [8]. Proximal injuries are more frequent than distal ones, and lesions closer to the ischial tuberosity generally require longer rehabilitation [8].

3.2.1 Clinical presentation and mechanisms of injury

Football players typically present with acute onset posterior thigh pain, often described as a sharp twinge, occurring during high-risk activities such as sprinting, kicking, or rapid deceleration [19, 35, 36]. Two main mechanisms have been identified [37, 38]:

- High-speed running mechanism: Eccentric contraction of the hamstrings during the terminal swing phase, especially against concentric quadriceps contraction. This most frequently involves the long head of the biceps femoris at the MTJ.
- Stretch-type mechanism: Extreme hip flexion with knee extension, as in a high kick, often involving the proximal semimembranosus tendon. These injuries are associated with longer recovery times due to free tendon involvement.

3.2.2 Physical examination

Assessment should follow a structured musculoskeletal protocol: inspection for swelling, ecchymosis, and muscle contour defects; palpation from origin to insertion; and evaluation of hip and knee range of motion. Strength testing is performed both concentrically (knee flexion at 90°) and eccentrically (near full extension), with foot rotation to bias specific hamstring muscles. When symptoms are atypical, neurologic examination and back/hip assessment are indicated to exclude other pathologies [35, 39, 40].

3.3 Nonoperative management

The immediate goals after a hamstring strain injury in footballers are rapid and safe RTP with minimal reinjury risk [34]. Treatment planning should begin with a precise structural diagnosis, identifying the muscle involved, the location of the lesion, and the tissue type (myofascial, MTJ, or intratendinous), as these factors influence prognosis and exercise selection [19, 34]. Intramuscular tendon involvement, particularly in the biceps femoris, tends to prolong rehabilitation and may alter management compared with typical MTJ injuries. In selected cases, this pattern may lead to surgical consideration [10].

Conservative care is primarily exercise-based, with emphasis on progressive loading under eccentric conditions. Eccentric knee-flexion training can improve RTP outcomes, although evidence on recurrence prevention is inconsistent [41]. In real-world football settings, early low-grade injuries may be under-recognized and undertreated, increasing the risk of subacute or chronic presentations [8].

Corticosteroid injections and oral nonsteroidal anti-inflammatory drugs (NSAIDs) are generally discouraged due to their potential negative impact on muscle healing and limited analgesic benefit in this setting [19]. Platelet-rich plasma (PRP) may be considered as an adjunct, particularly in younger professionals with severe hamstring strain injury, but current evidence is insufficient and protocols vary widely [19].

Despite widespread use, no universal rehabilitation algorithm exists, and comparative evidence across protocols is sparse. Structural patterns such as intratendinous lesions often require longer recovery and, in certain cases, may ultimately warrant surgical repair [34].

3.4 Surgical indications

In professional football players, surgery is primarily indicated when the structural damage is such that nonoperative management is unlikely to restore full function or enable a safe return to preinjury performance [12].

The most frequent indications include complete proximal avulsions or total tendon ruptures, osseous avulsion fractures, myotendinous lesions with complete loss of continuity at the musculotendinous junction, and full-thickness muscle belly tears with significant retraction, commonly considered relevant when ≥2 cm in high-demand athletes. Persistent pain or functional limitations following an adequate, criterion-based rehabilitation trial for partial injuries may also warrant surgical consideration [42, 43]. Additionally, imaging evidence of incomplete healing, such as persistent fluid between the ischial tuberosity and tendon footprint, despite optimal conservative care, and intramuscular tendon injuries with prolonged recovery or recurrent dysfunction in elite players, are recognized indications for operative repair [44].

In chronic settings, surgery may be justified in the presence of painful calcified avulsion remnants, myositis ossificans, adhesions involving the sciatic nerve, or significant muscular deficits unresponsive to structured rehabilitation. For such cases, surgical objectives extend beyond anatomical restoration to include relief of pain, recovery of strength, and prevention of further neurological compromise.

Timing is a key prognostic factor. Comparative studies show that acute repair (≤6 weeks; mean 2.8 weeks) is associated with higher satisfaction rates (95% vs. 77%), greater likelihood of return to the same competitive level (92% vs. 85%), and shorter time to RTP (4.5 vs. 5.6 months) compared with chronic repair (mean 46 weeks) [12]. Complication rates are also lower with early intervention (13.95 vs. 25.00%), including fewer neurological sequelae (1.66 vs. 9.04%) [12]. The overall evidence favors timely surgical repair in athletes when indicated [12].

3.5 Surgical technique

The anatomical region of the hamstrings is the most complex among those discussed in this chapter. The complexity lies in the fact that, while in the adductors the main focus is on a single tendon and in the rectus femoris on a muscle belly with two tendons, in this case, the ischial insertion involves three tendons. The long head of the biceps femoris and the semitendinosus insert together as a conjoined tendon, posterior and distal to the insertion of the semimembranosus. The tendon of the latter passes medially and beneath the conjoined tendon, crossing it to insert laterally and slightly superiorly on the ischium.

From a surgical perspective, lesions in this area may present with large hematomas, significant tendon or myotendinous gaps (up to 15–18 cm), and involvement of the sciatic nerve, which is located very close to the region. In such cases, the incision may be longitudinal along the course of the retracted tendon when a large gap is present or transverse under the gluteal fold, more commonly for chronic tendinopathies or in cases with smaller gaps. In either approach, access to the ischium requires partial release of some fibers of the gluteus maximus, which are repaired at the end of the procedure.

As described in previous sections, the tendon is often not anatomically normal but thickened due to chronic tendinopathy, making tendon revision necessary before reinsertion or repair. Frequently, sciatic nerve release is also required after identification, due to adhesions that may have formed. In acute hamstring lesions, large hematomas are commonly encountered, which help localize the injury site and create space to mobilize and retension the retracted tendon-muscle unit. In the absence of hematoma and in chronic lesions evaluated more than 1 month after trauma, it may be impossible to restore the tendon to its original footprint because of scar repair involving adjacent muscles and retraction of the injured tendon and muscle.

When reinsertion is performed, the bone at the ischial insertion must be prepared by curettage, and one or two anchors, either titanium or polyether ether ketone (PEEK), are applied. High-strength, nonabsorbable sutures are then used to retension and secure the tendon back to its anatomical footprint, with the knee flexed. Intraoperative flexion-extension maneuvers are performed to confirm the stability of the repair. Careful hemostasis is required to avoid postoperative hematomas, and wound closure is performed in layers. The skin is closed with barbed sutures to reduce the risk of subcutaneous granulomas from knots, followed by the application of Steri-Strips and usually a compressive dressing. Drains are not placed.

Figures 1 and **2** show a case of proximal biceps femoris injury treated surgically. **Figure 3** illustrates a case of distal biceps femoris injury treated surgically.

3.6 Postoperative rehabilitation

After surgery, the patient is positioned supine with the knee slightly flexed, supported by a pillow. It is recommended to avoid hip flexion with the knee extended for a period determined by the surgeon. Passive mobilization of the hip and knee begins the day after surgery, and the patient is allowed partial weight-bearing with crutches for the first 15 days, followed by gradual weaning. Once the sutures are removed, a rehabilitation program is initiated, focusing on strengthening the thigh musculature to protect the hamstring muscles. After 3 weeks, selective isometric strengthening can be introduced, progressing to eccentric strengthening at 6 weeks.

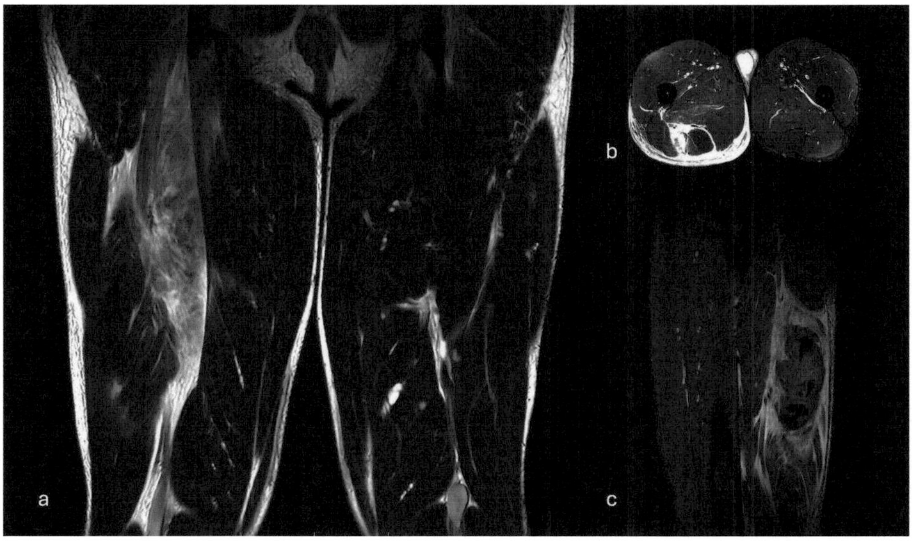

Figure 1.
MRI of the right thigh performed 4 days after trauma in a 36-year-old professional football player, showing a complete grade 3 lesion of the proximal myotendinous junction of the biceps femoris with tendon retraction >12 cm. A pseudohematocyst of approximately 10 × 2.5 cm is evident at the lesion site, associated with diffuse perilesional edema extending to adjacent muscle fascicles. (a) Coronal view, (b) Axial view, (c) Sagittal view.

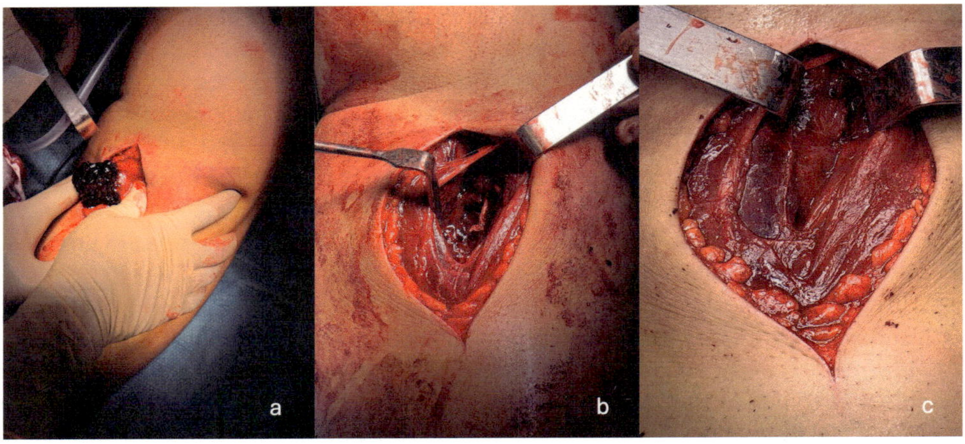

Figure 2.
Intraoperative images of the patient presented in **Figure 1**, *with a lesion of the proximal myotendinous junction of the biceps femoris and tendon retraction: (a) hematoma evacuation; (b) tendon retraction; (c) tendon retensioning.*

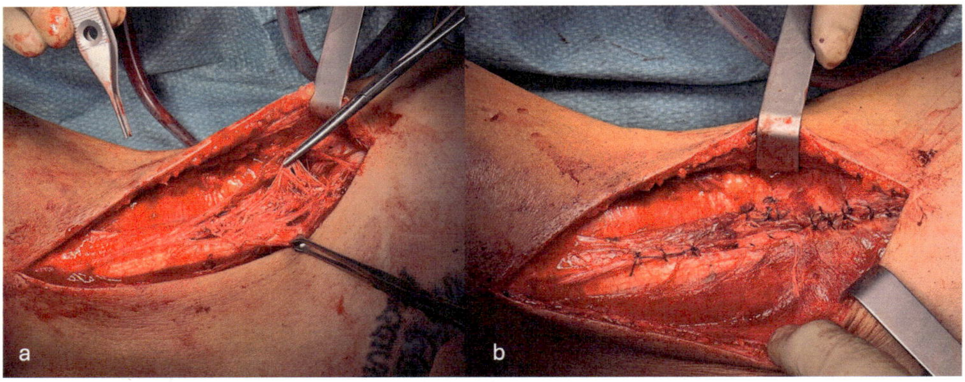

Figure 3.
Distal biceps femoris myotendinous lesion in a 31-year-old professional football player. Intraoperative images: (a) lesion, (b) suture with tendon retensioning.

In cases of hamstring reinsertion, running is typically postponed until 2 months after surgery, later than in adductor or rectus femoris repairs. Sport-specific exercises follow, and full recovery is generally expected between four and 6 months, depending on the extent of the lesion.

4. Adductor injuries

The anatomy and biomechanics of the adductor are reported in Appendix B.

4.1 Epidemiology and risk factors in professional football

The true incidence of adductor injuries in football is difficult to determine, as minor strains often go unreported and lesions may occur within complex groin pathologies [45]. In general athletic cohorts, adductor strains represent about 10%

of all sports injuries and a major proportion of groin lesions [46]. In football, groin injuries account for 10–18% of all reported cases in men, with female incidence around 9–13% [46].

Longitudinal data from 15 professional seasons (2000–2015) identified 671 adductor injuries, with no baseline differences compared to matched controls. The mean age at injury was 26.0 ± 3.8 years for attackers, 26.9 ± 3.9 for midfielders, and 26.5 ± 3.8 for defenders, while goalkeepers were older (29.0 ± 3.3 years, $P < .001$) [47].

Key risk factors include reduced adductor strength, low adductor-abductor strength ratio, previous adductor injury, restricted hip mobility, leg length discrepancy, and dominant kicking leg [46, 48, 49]. Fatigue, inadequate conditioning, and insufficient warm-up also contribute [48]. The high eccentric loads during kicking, rapid changes of direction, and decelerations in football place considerable strain on the adductor complex, increasing the risk of recurrence, particularly in older players and those with prior groin injuries [48].

4.2 Clinical assessment

Early and precise diagnosis of adductor injuries is essential to guide treatment and minimize time loss, but prognosis may be challenging due to the variability in injury grade, anatomical location, and mechanism [45, 46, 50]. In professional football, recurrent injuries and underdiagnosed low-grade strains remain significant issues [46].

4.2.1 Clinical presentation and mechanisms of injury

Adductor muscle and tendon injuries typically present with acute or progressive medial thigh or groin pain, often triggered by high-risk activities such as sprinting, rapid change of direction, kicking, or forced hip abduction [45, 46, 50, 51]. Mechanisms are generally classified as [46, 51]:

- Open-chain: kicking, jumping;
- Closed-chain: cutting, reaching, or acceleration–deceleration maneuvers;
- Direct trauma: contusion from a ball, opponent, or equipment;
- Eccentric overload: forced hip abduction during adduction, potentially causing tendon avulsion.

Chronic tendinopathy usually develops over weeks to months due to repetitive loading without adequate recovery, often exacerbated by biomechanical factors such as hip external rotation, genu valgus, or excessive pronation during gait [51].

4.2.2 Physical examination

Assessment should follow a systematic hip and groin protocol [50]:

- Inspection for swelling, ecchymosis, and contour changes, including delayed bruising tracking distally;
- Gait observation for Trendelenburg or coxalgic patterns;

- Palpation from the origin to insertion of the adductors, including the pubic ramus, adductor longus origin, and adjacent structures, to detect focal tenderness, defects, or hematomas;

- Strength testing with resisted hip adduction, inside straight leg lift, and passive stretching;

- Functional testing of abdominal muscles and iliopsoas to detect combined injuries;

- Range of motion assessment for hip and knee, with bilateral comparison.

When the presentation is atypical, non-musculoskeletal causes (inguinal hernia, abdominal or genitourinary pathology) should be excluded through targeted examination.

4.3 Nonoperative management

Conservative treatment represents the cornerstone of initial care for adductor muscle and tendon injuries. The early phase follows the established principles of soft-tissue management (protection, optimal loading, ice, compression, and elevation) [52]. Resting in a supported supine position with slight hip flexion or the use of crutches may reduce tension on the injured structures. Cryotherapy and compression with elastic bandages or sleeves help to control bleeding and pain in the first 48 hours.

Analgesics and NSAIDs may provide symptomatic relief, although their potential impact on healing requires cautious use [52]. Physiotherapy usually begins after 48–72 hours, once acute bleeding has subsided. Initial interventions aim to reduce inflammation and protective spasm, followed by progressive mobilization, motor control retraining, and strengthening across the kinetic chain [45].

Rehabilitation programs should be adapted to the grade and location of injury. Eccentric strengthening, proprioceptive exercises, and functional drills are essential, but the load must be carefully titrated: discomfort during exercise is acceptable, while significant pain during or after training indicates overload and requires adjustment. Particular attention should be given to associated deficits in posture or movement patterns, which often predispose to recurrence [53–55].

RTP decisions are guided by clinical criteria rather than imaging. The athlete should demonstrate pain-free adductor contraction, tolerance to sport-specific drills (sprinting, cutting, and agility testing), and adequate functional stability. Structured, criteria-based rehabilitation appears more effective in reducing reinjury than protocols based solely on MRI grading [56].

Chronic adductor-related pain often requires a modified conservative approach. Many athletes, particularly in team sports such as football or ice hockey, continue to compete during the season while undergoing maintenance physiotherapy, functional training, and external support (sleeves, wraps, or taping). However, definitive resolution is frequently delayed until off-season recovery [49].

Despite widespread use, nonoperative management has limitations. Persistent pain beyond 3 months despite adherence to rehabilitation, or lack of functional recovery, should prompt orthopedic referral [57]. In addition, some structural patterns, such as complete avulsions or advanced tendinopathy, may not respond adequately to conservative treatment and progress to surgical indication [58, 59].

4.4 Surgical indications

Surgery for adductor injuries is relatively uncommon, but it plays an important role in selected cases. Clear indications include complete avulsions of the adductor longus origin, high-grade (grade 3) tears with loss of function, or chronic tendinopathy unresponsive to at least 3 months of structured rehabilitation [58, 59]. Avulsion injuries, particularly when bone fragments are involved, require timely referral. Reinsertion is generally indicated when the diastasis exceeds 0.5 cm, particularly in association with a bony fragment.

Early intervention is advised because delayed surgery is complicated by tendon retraction and scarring, which increase technical difficulty and compromise outcomes [57].

In professional athletes, surgery is also considered when functional performance is significantly impaired or when combined lesions are present, such as sports hernia or osteitis pubis [46]. Chronic groin pain often reveals a spectrum of pathologies at surgical exploration, underscoring the importance of referral to experienced surgeons [46].

Timing is crucial: surgery is ideally performed within days for acute avulsions, before retraction and scarring occur. In chronic cases, delayed surgery can still be beneficial but often demands more extensive dissection and carries a higher risk.

Nonoperative management remains the first-line approach for most adductor injuries, while surgery is reserved for complete avulsions, severe tendon ruptures, or chronic cases refractory to structured rehabilitation. The decision should consider injury severity, functional demands, stage of the competitive season, and the athlete's goals, balancing early RTP with long-term durability of function.

4.5 Surgical technique

The anatomy of the inguinal region is complex, since avulsion of the adductor longus (by far the most frequent) is often not the only structure that requires repair. This is because the adductor longus is part of the pyramidal-anterior pubic ligament-adductor longus complex (PLAC). In chronic or recurrent lesions, anatomical alterations may be present, leading to a different surgical scenario compared to acute injuries.

The incision is made in the medial region of the hip, guided by palpation of the adductor longus tendon. After opening the subcutaneous tissue, the surgeon reaches the fascia of the adductor longus, which is often thickened and adherent to the underlying tissues due to initial attempts at spontaneous repair. This occurs because there is usually a time interval of 10–20 days between the traumatic event, clinical and imaging assessment, and the organization of surgery. During this time, fibrous scar tissue begins to form.

If the tendon shows preexisting insertional degeneration, which is common in athletes practicing sports with frequent changes of direction, such as soccer, the tissue must be carefully dissected, the proximal portion scarified, and sometimes reinforced with resorbable sutures to restore its shape and allow proper tension. Before reinsertion, the tendon must also be mobilized distally. If a rigid tendon adherent to surrounding tissues is reattached, the risk of recurrence is high due to excessive tension. Indeed, tenotomy procedures are sometimes performed for excessive tension in insertional tendinopathies.

Once prepared, the pubic tubercle is identified, debrided of residual tissue, and, in some cases, microperforated to stimulate healing. The site is then prepared for the anchor, which can be titanium or biomaterials such as PEEK. The anchor or screw is fixed into the bone, its stability is tested by pulling the high-resistance sutures, and then it is used with needles to secure and retension the tendon. Reinsertion is performed with the hip in adduction, and subsequent abduction maneuvers are carried out to test stability before reconstructing the overlying layers. Accurate hemostasis is essential to reduce the risk of postoperative hematomas. Drains are not usually placed. Skin closure is typically performed with intradermal self-locking sutures to avoid unaesthetic scars, prevent subcutaneous knots that may form granulomas, and improve wound sealing in a region at risk of infection due to local sweating. Steri-Strips and medicated dressings are applied.

In this region, direct repair of myotendinous lesions is more challenging because they are less common, though possible. Sometimes post-traumatic hematomas must be evacuated. In cases of recurrent lesions, it may be necessary to remove painful calcifications, which are sometimes mobile, and repair the underlying tissue. In this surgical field, complications such as infection, wound dehiscence, or mobilization of the implanted anchor are relatively more frequent.

Figure 4 presents a case of adductor injury treated surgically.

4.6 Postoperative rehabilitation

The patient can begin early mobilization of the hip, avoiding flexion beyond 60° for the first 15 days and refraining from passive or active abduction and active adduction during the first 2 weeks. Partial weight-bearing with two crutches is allowed during this initial phase. After suture removal, usually around day 15, full weight-bearing may be resumed, and aquatic rehabilitation can be initiated.

Strengthening of the surrounding hip musculature can start early, while specific isometric exercises for the adductors are introduced at approximately 3 weeks, together with stationary cycling and progressive cross-training. At 4 weeks, light running can be initiated. After 5 weeks, eccentric strengthening is progressively included, followed by sport-specific drills and gradual reintroduction to running after 8 weeks.

In most cases, a complete return to competitive sports is expected within 3–4 months, provided that strength and neuromuscular control testing are satisfactory. Follow-up assessments are typically performed with an ultrasound during rehabilitation. Routine postoperative MRI is not indicated.

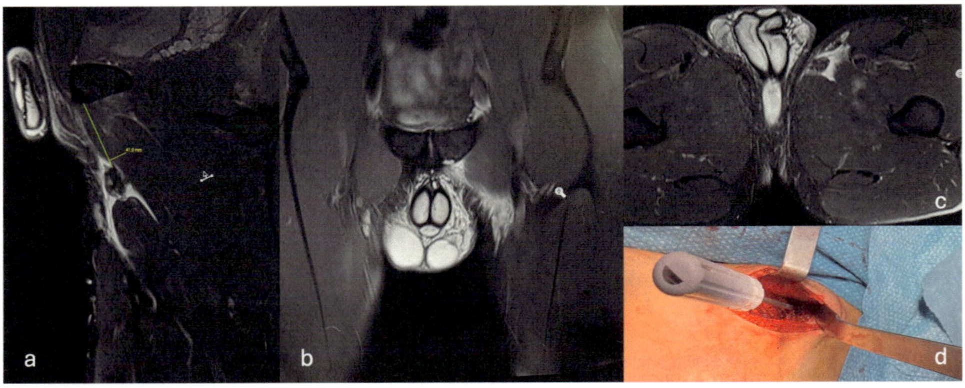

Figure 4.
Adductor injury: MRI images (a) sagittal view, (b) coronal view, (c) axial view, and tendon reinsertion with anchor (d).

5. Quadriceps injuries

The anatomy and biomechanics of the quadriceps are reported in Appendix C.

5.1 Epidemiology and risk factors in professional football

Quadriceps injuries are the third most common muscle injuries in football, after hamstring and adductor lesions, but they often result in longer time loss [11]. They account for about 5% of all football injuries and nearly 20% of muscle-tendon injuries, with the rectus femoris being the muscle most frequently affected, particularly in its proximal and distal thirds [11, 60]. These injuries typically occur during sprinting, kicking, or jumping, when the rectus femoris undergoes forceful eccentric contractions [11, 60]. Direct traumas, such as contusions sustained during tackles, are also frequent, especially involving the vastus intermedius, lateralis, and medialis, and are often described as "dead leg" injuries [11].

Although quadriceps contusions are also common in contact sports such as rugby, American football, and ice hockey, football presents a particularly high risk. Large prospective studies in European elite clubs show that most quadriceps injuries are mild to moderate muscle tears [27]. Fatigue plays a central role, with most injuries occurring in the later stages of matches [61].

The main risk factor is a previous quadriceps injury, with a recurrence rate particularly high in the rectus femoris due to its high proportion of type II fibers, which are prone to eccentric overload and fatigue [60, 62]. Additional factors include leg dominance, with a higher incidence in the dominant kicking leg; asymmetries in strength or flexibility between quadriceps and hamstrings; surface conditions such as dry playing fields; and insufficient recovery during competition, where the risk of injury may be up to 25 times higher than in training [11, 63].

Unlike tendon ruptures, which increase with age, quadriceps muscle strains do not appear to be age-dependent [64]. Instead, the main determinants are workload, fatigue, and sport-specific demands, making football a particularly challenging context for quadriceps injury prevention.

5.2 Clinical assessment

A thorough clinical assessment of quadriceps injuries is essential to differentiate between strains, contusions, tendinopathies, and ruptures, as each condition has specific mechanisms and clinical features that guide management.

5.2.1 Clinical presentation and mechanisms of injury

Quadriceps strains are typically caused by sudden eccentric contractions during activities such as sprinting, jumping, or kicking. Symptoms range from mild discomfort to severe pain, often accompanied by swelling or ecchymosis. Patients may report a "pop" or tightness at the time of injury, with the rectus femoris being the most frequently affected, especially at the central tendon or myotendinous junctions [60].

Contusions result from direct trauma, producing localized tenderness, swelling, and sometimes hematomas. Severity is graded by preserved knee flexion (>90° mild, 45–90° moderate, <45° severe). Complications include myositis ossificans in severe or untreated cases [65].

Quadriceps tendinopathy, though less frequent than patellar tendinopathy, develops through repetitive overuse, causing anterior knee pain and tenderness near the superior patella or anterior inferior iliac spine. It often impairs resisted knee extension or hip flexion [66].

Tendon ruptures usually occur during explosive movements and present with sudden, sharp pain, swelling, and loss of knee extension. A palpable defect proximal to the patella is typical of quadriceps tendon rupture [67, 68].

Structurally, rectus femoris injuries can affect the proximal tendons, central septum, or distal myotendinous junction. Proximal lesions weaken hip flexion, distal ones compromise knee extension, and chronic central tendon ruptures may mimic soft-tissue masses [69, 70].

5.2.2 Physical examination

Examination should focus on inspection, palpation, and functional testing. Visible swelling, ecchymosis, or thigh asymmetry suggests significant injury, while tendon ruptures often reveal a palpable gap.

Strength testing of knee extension and hip flexion helps grade the injury: grade I (minimal tearing, preserved strength), grade II (partial tear, reduced strength), and grade III (complete tear, functional loss) [11]. In contusions, prognosis can be estimated by knee flexion range of motion, which correlates with severity [65].

Lesion location influences clinical signs: proximal injuries impair hip flexion, while mid- and distal lesions reduce knee extension. Even in severe ruptures, hematomas may be minimal, and chronic central tendon injuries can resemble soft-tissue tumors [11].

5.3 Nonoperative management

Most quadriceps injuries are treated conservatively, in line with the general principles of muscle injury management. The healing process is classically divided into three overlapping phases: muscle fiber degeneration and inflammation (1–3 days), regeneration (3–4 weeks), and maturation with remodeling (3–6 months) [11].

In the acute stage, the standard approach is protection, rest, ice, compression, and elevation, aiming to reduce bleeding, swelling, and pain [11]. Cryotherapy is safe and helps lower tissue metabolism, while elevation and compression limit edema. Severe strains may require temporary non-weight-bearing with crutches. Early initiation of passive range of motion, especially gentle knee flexion, together with isometric contractions when tolerated, is encouraged to maintain mobility and prevent atrophy, although high-quality evidence remains limited [11].

Quadriceps contusions require similar management, but immobilization of the knee in 120° flexion during the first 24 hours has been shown to reduce recovery time [71]. Once pain subsides, progressive stretching and strengthening are introduced. Rehabilitation progresses gradually from passive and active mobilization to isometric, eccentric, and gym-based exercises before advancing to field-specific training [65]. The key is a controlled and pain-free progression to minimize the risk of reinjury and avoid compensatory motor patterns [65].

NSAIDs may be used for short courses, although evidence of their benefit is limited, and some concerns exist regarding delayed healing [71].

RTP decisions remain complex, but consensus exists that athletes should demonstrate complete symptom resolution, full recovery of strength and function, and pass sport-specific functional testing before medical clearance [11, 72].

5.4 Surgical indications

Surgical treatment is reserved for specific and severe injuries. Complete quadriceps or patellar tendon ruptures, as well as high-grade partial ruptures, clearly require operative repair [73]. Similarly, cases with massive hematoma and suspicion of acute compartment syndrome warrant urgent surgical evaluation [11].

In elite athletes, operative management can also be considered for proximal rectus femoris avulsions with retraction >2 cm, recurrent proximal tendon injuries, and central tendon ruptures—especially in chronic or recurrent cases [11]. Surgical exploration may also be indicated in unstable myotendinous junction tears, severe insertional lesions, or when hematoma evacuation is required.

The goals of surgery are to restore normal anatomy, reinforce tendon structure when needed, and reduce recurrence risk, while maintaining minimal complication rates [11]. Reported outcomes suggest a favorable return to preinjury performance, with postoperative return-to-play typically expected within 3–5 months, depending on the extent of repair [11, 73].

5.5 Surgical technique

The insertional anatomy of the rectus femoris is complex, and well-recognized anatomical variants exist. The surgical decision must take into account several factors, including the classification of the lesion, the presence of recurrence, the gap between the insertion site and the remaining tendon, and possible involvement of the myotendinous junction. The skin incision is made longitudinally, centered over the rectus femoris tendon, and extended up to 3 cm from its proximal insertion, which can then be easily exposed. The dissection proceeds by creating a plane between the sartorius and the tensor fasciae latae, as in the anterior hip approach, by incising the overlying fascia. The myotendinous junction of the rectus femoris is then reached and followed proximally to its insertion.

The tendon in this region is often thickened, degenerated, and calcified, particularly in cases of recurrent tears or chronic tendinopathy that have subsequently ruptured. At this point, the gap can be identified, which may occur between the tendon and the bone, within the intermediate portion of the tendon, or at the myotendinous junction, with clear retraction of the muscle belly, often described in imaging as a rounded myotendinous retraction of the muscle belly. The tendon must be scarified with longitudinal incisions, degenerated tissue and calcifications removed, and reinforced or repaired with the remaining stump. Reinsertion into the pelvis is performed using a titanium or PEEK anchor or screw, since end-to-end sutures of proximal tears usually provide insufficient strength. The bone is prepared with microperforations to stimulate healing before anchor placement. The anchor, with high-resistance nonabsorbable sutures, is then used to secure the tendon. In cases involving the conjoined tendon, an anchor can be placed in the intermediate region between the direct and indirect rectus femoris tendons. Reinsertion must be carried out with the hip flexed, followed by dynamic mobilization tests to verify stability.

During the approach, care must be taken to protect the lateral femoral cutaneous nerve in order to avoid temporary or permanent sensory deficits of the anterolateral thigh. Accurate hemostasis is crucial to prevent postoperative hematomas. Closure proceeds in layers, suturing the fascia between the sartorius and tensor fasciae latae, followed by subcutaneous tissue and skin using an intradermal barbed suture, to avoid knots that may cause granulomas. Steri-Strips and a medicated dressing are then applied. Drains are not used.

Complications of rectus femoris repair include local calcifications, hematomas, and recurrent tears. At this site, the risk of surgical site infection is lower compared with adductor repairs.

In cases of myotendinous junction lesions, particular attention must be paid to repairing the area with nonabsorbable sutures and avoiding excessive tension. For such lesions, postoperative recovery is slower due to the inherent difficulty of suturing muscle to the remaining tendon, given the poor mechanical resistance of muscle tissue. Finally, in cases of mid-tendon tears with a large residual gap, a "bridging suture" technique can be used, reinforced by repairing adjacent muscle tissue to improve vascularization. This approach has demonstrated the capacity to promote tendon repair and regeneration over time.

Figures 5 and **6** show a case of rectus femoris injury treated surgically.

5.6 Postoperative rehabilitation

The patient is discharged on the first postoperative day. Hip mobilization is allowed, with flexion not exceeding 90° during the first month. Hip extension should

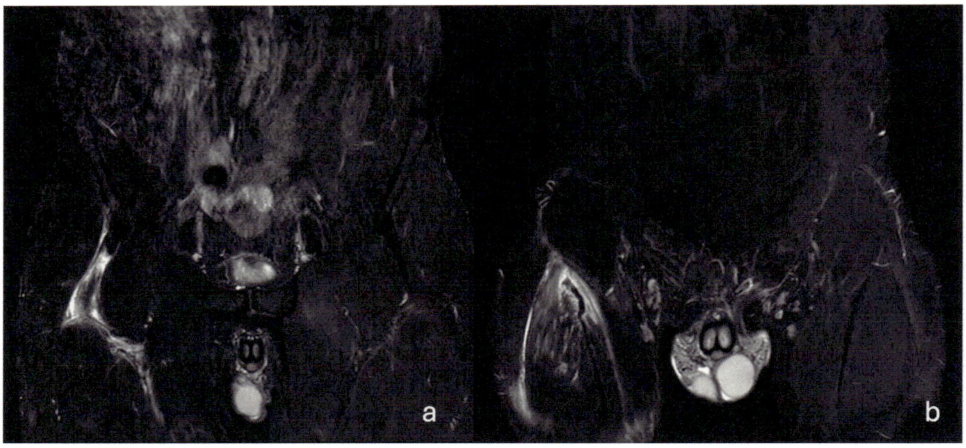

Figure 5.
MRI of the right thigh in a 34-year-old professional football player, showing a complete rectus femoris lesion. (a) and (b) Coronal views.

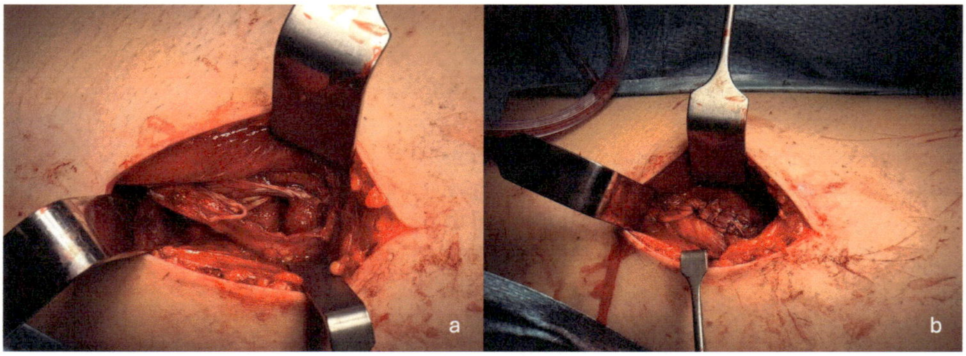

Figure 6.
Intraoperative images of the patient shown in **Figure 5***: (a) lesion, (b) suture with tendon retensioning.*

be avoided, while adduction, abduction, and gentle rotational movements are permitted. The use of two crutches is recommended for the first 2 weeks, after which sutures can be removed and a rehabilitation program aimed at strengthening the periarticular hip musculature to protect the rectus femoris can begin.

Gentle isometric activation of the rectus femoris is allowed after 3 weeks. Running may be resumed after approximately 40 days, depending on local conditions and the type of repair performed. In cases of myotendinous repairs or tendon repairs with large gaps, this protocol should be delayed.

At 6 weeks, eccentric strengthening exercises are initiated. After 2 months, progressive field-based rehabilitation begins, including sport-specific exercises of gradually increasing intensity. Full recovery is typically expected within 4 months.

6. Reinjury

Reinjury of thigh tendons, particularly the rectus femoris and hamstrings, remains one of the most challenging scenarios in sports medicine. Recurrent lesions not only prolong recovery and limit performance but may also compromise an athlete's career. While most primary injuries can be managed conservatively, the recurrence of tendon injuries often shifts the balance toward surgical treatment, especially in professional athletes, where rapid and durable RTP is essential [13].

6.1 Hamstring reinjury

Hamstring reinjuries are common, particularly when the central tendon or the distal MTJ of the biceps femoris is involved [12]. Recurrence rates in this region may exceed 50%, and surgical management is often necessary when conservative care fails [74]. Surgical indications in hamstring reinjuries include:

- Symptomatic but stable lesions resistant to medical and physical therapy, often with persistent pain during sport-specific actions;

- Hamstring syndrome, characterized by sciatic nerve irritation and recurrent functional limitation;

- Multiple recurrences despite adequate rehabilitation and progressive RTP protocols;

- Structural complications, such as calcifications or large fibrotic scars, that alter tendon biomechanics.

Surgical intervention in these cases typically aims to restore tendon continuity, decompress neural structures if needed, and prevent further recurrence. Acute repair has shown superior outcomes compared with delayed surgery, with higher RTP rates and fewer complications [75].

6.2 Adductor reinjury

Adductor longus injuries are common in sports requiring rapid directional changes, such as football and ice hockey, and recurrent lesions may compromise performance and lead to chronic groin pain [13]. While the majority of first injuries are successfully managed conservatively, recurrent or chronic cases pose a greater challenge.

Surgical intervention for adductor reinjuries is considered in the following scenarios [12]:

- Persistent pain with a stable but symptomatic lesion, refractory to medical and physical therapy;
- Multiple reinjuries despite an adequate rehabilitation process;
- Complications such as calcifications, chronic tendinopathy, or fibrotic scarring alter tendon biomechanics and increase recurrence risk;
- Associated PLAC complex involvement, where anatomical disruption prevents spontaneous healing.

Surgery usually consists of tendon release, debridement of fibrotic tissue or calcifications, and, when feasible, reattachment of the adductor longus to the pubic tubercle with suture anchors. Accurate tensioning of the tendon during reattachment is essential to avoid excessive strain, which predisposes to further recurrence.

6.3 Quadriceps reinjury

The rectus femoris is highly exposed to reinjury due to its dual origin and long intramuscular tendon. Central tendon involvement significantly increases recurrence risk and delays RTP [12]. Surgery is generally considered in specific scenarios:

- Persistent pain despite adequate conservative management, with stable but symptomatic lesions.
- Multiple reinjuries following structured rehabilitation programs suggest underlying tendon degeneration or biomechanical vulnerability.
- Complications such as calcifications or fibrotic remodeling impair tendon elasticity and healing.

In these cases, surgical repair or reinforcement of the affected tendon may restore mechanical integrity and reduce the likelihood of further recurrence [11].

6.4 Clinical implications

Reinjury of thigh tendons represents a major clinical challenge. While most cases can be managed conservatively, surgery becomes indicated in specific scenarios: persistent painful lesions resistant to medical and physical therapy, multiple recurrences despite adequate rehabilitation, and complications such as calcifications.

In the rectus femoris, surgery is also considered for chronic or recurrent lesions involving the central tendon. In the hamstrings, surgical repair may be required in recurrent proximal avulsions, hamstring syndrome, or symptomatic tendon retraction. For the adductors, surgery is reserved for recurrent avulsions or chronic painful lesions unresponsive to conservative care.

Careful patient selection, accurate imaging, and individualized rehabilitation are key to improving outcomes and minimizing recurrence.

7. Conclusions

Thigh tendon injuries in professional football remain a major clinical and performance challenge. While most cases recover with conservative management, surgery is warranted for complete avulsions, symptomatic lesions resistant to rehabilitation, and recurrent injuries complicated by tendon degeneration or calcifications. Central tendon involvement in the rectus femoris and hamstrings, as well as adductor avulsions, are particularly prone to recurrence and may benefit from timely surgical repair. Accurate diagnosis, early recognition of high-risk lesions, and structured rehabilitation protocols are essential to reduce reinjury rates. Personalized treatment strategies, integrating imaging, surgical expertise, and tailored rehabilitation, are key to ensuring safe return to play and long-term durability of function.

Conflict of interest

The authors declare no conflict of interest regarding the contents of this chapter.

Appendices A. Hamstring injuries

A.1 Anatomy and biomechanics

The hamstring muscle complex occupies the posterior compartment of the thigh and consists of three primary muscles: the biceps femoris, semitendinosus, and semimembranosus [76]. These muscles play an essential role in activities ranging from upright stance to explosive movements such as sprinting, jumping, and rapid changes in direction [76].

1. Origins and insertions

The biceps femoris has two distinct heads:

- Long head: originates from the ischial tuberosity and inserts into the fibular head and lateral tibial condyle [76];
- Short head: originates from the lateral lip of the femoral linea aspera and inserts into the fibular head and lateral tibial condyle [76].

The semitendinosus arises from the medial aspect of the ischial tuberosity and inserts on the medial surface of the tibia at the pes anserinus [76].

The semimembranosus originates from the ischial tuberosity and inserts into the medial tibial condyle [76].

2. Innervation and vascular supply

Innervation is provided by the sciatic nerve, formed by contributions from the lower lumbar and upper sacral plexuses. The nerve emerges through the greater sciatic foramen and descends along the posterior thigh, bifurcating at the knee into the tibial and common peroneal (fibular) nerves [77].

- The tibial nerve supplies the semimembranosus, semitendinosus, and long head of the biceps femoris.

- The common peroneal nerve innervates the short head of the biceps femoris.

The vascular supply is derived from perforating branches of the deep femoral artery (profunda femoris) [77, 78]. Venous drainage parallels the arterial system, and lymphatic drainage follows similar pathways, ultimately reaching the lumbar lymphatic trunks and cisterna chyli [77, 78].

3. Relevant anatomical relationships

The close proximity of the sciatic nerve to the hamstring muscles explains the potential for radicular symptoms following hamstring injuries (**Figure 7**) [35, 36, 39]. Distally, the hamstrings define the borders of the popliteal fossa: the biceps femoris laterally and the semitendinosus and semimembranosus medially [79].

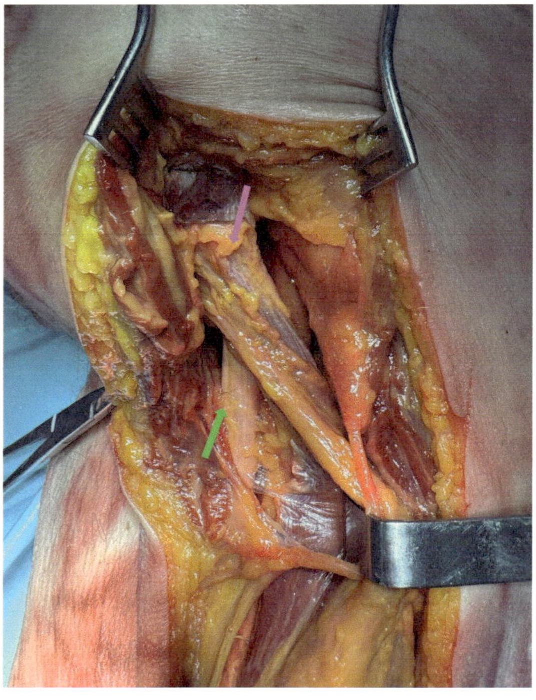

Figure 7.
Cadaveric image showing the close anatomical relationship between the sciatic nerve (green arrow) and the conjoined tendon of the hamstrings at its insertion on the ischial tuberosity (purple arrow).

4. Anatomical variants

Although uncommon, anatomical variations have been described, including separate tendinous origins for the semitendinosus and long head of the biceps femoris, an accessory third head of the biceps femoris, or even bilateral absence of the semimembranosus [15, 80, 81]. Such variants can have clinical implications, particularly in anterior cruciate ligament reconstruction, where hamstring autografts are frequently used [81]. Additionally, anatomical alterations may predispose to common peroneal nerve entrapment, most often at the level of the fibular head [82].

5. Biomechanics and function

With the exception of the short head of the biceps femoris, most hamstring muscles span both the hip and knee joints [83]. Their primary actions are knee flexion and hip extension [83].

The biceps femoris contributes to external rotation of the hip and tibia (with the knee flexed), whereas the semitendinosus and semimembranosus contribute to internal rotation [83].

Functionally, the hamstrings are critical for deceleration during running, directional changes, and kicking. This is achieved through eccentric contractions that slow the forward swing of the limb during the terminal swing phase of gait [33, 84, 85]. They also act as dynamic stabilizers of the knee, working synergistically with the anterior cruciate ligament to limit anterior tibial translation during heel strike [15].

Appendices B. Adductor injuries

B.1 Anatomy and biomechanics

The hip adductor muscle group occupies the medial compartment of the thigh, positioned between the quadriceps anteriorly and the hamstring muscles posteriorly. It extends from the inferior pelvis to the femur, with the gracilis being the only muscle to cross the knee and insert on the proximal medial tibia [86, 87]. This group shapes the medial contour of the thigh and includes the adductor magnus, adductor longus, adductor brevis, gracilis, pectineus, and, variably, the adductor minimus [86, 88].

1. Origins and insertions

The adductor magnus originates from the inferior pubic ramus, ischial ramus, and ischial tuberosity, dividing into two functional portions [89, 90]:

- The adductor (pubofemoral) portion inserts along the linea aspera and medial supracondylar line, merging with the short head of the biceps femoris proximally, thereby contributing to femoral and pelvic stability.
- The hamstring (ischiocondylar) portion runs vertically from the ischial tuberosity to the adductor tubercle on the medial femoral condyle.

The adductor longus originates from the superior pubic ramus and pubic symphysis, inserting on the linea aspera and forming distally part of the vasto-adductor membrane [90].

The adductor brevis arises from the inferior pubic ramus and inserts on the proximal linea aspera [90].

The adductor minimus, when present, is a proximal lateral separation of the adductor magnus, extending from the inferior pubic ramus to the linea aspera [90].

The pectineus runs from the superior pubic ramus to the pectineal line and proximal linea aspera [90].

The gracilis originates from the inferior border of the pubic symphysis and inserts on the superficial pes anserinus of the tibia [90].

2. Innervation and vascular supply

The obturator nerve (L2–L4) supplies most of the adductor compartment, except for the pectineus, which receives innervation from the femoral nerve, and the hamstring portion of the adductor magnus, which is innervated by the tibial division of the sciatic nerve [89, 90]. Anatomical studies have demonstrated dual innervation of the distal adductor magnus by both the posterior division of the obturator nerve and the tibial portion of the sciatic nerve in over 90% of specimens [91].

The vascular supply derives from the obturator artery, perforating branches of the profunda femoris, and the medial femoral circumflex artery, with distal contributions from the femoral, popliteal, and genicular arteries [90]. Lymphatic drainage is directed to the deep inguinal lymph nodes.

3. Relevant anatomical relationships

The proximal adductor origin integrates with the pyramidalis-anterior pubic ligament-adductor longus complex (PLAC), a functional unit involved in proximal tendon avulsions [92].

The adductor canal (Hunter's canal), located between the adductor magnus, adductor longus, and vastus medialis, contains the femoral artery, vein, and saphenous nerve and is partly covered by the vasto-adductor membrane [90]. Distally, the adductor hiatus in the inferior segment of the adductor magnus allows the femoral vessels to pass into the popliteal fossa [89].

4. Anatomical variants

Variations include the presence of a distinct or partially fused adductor minimus, absence of the minimus with inferior extension of the quadratus femoris, and the presence of a vasto-adductor membrane, which can occasionally compress the femoral artery [88, 93]. Morphological differences in fiber arrangement between proximal and distal segments of the adductor magnus may influence its stabilizing versus mobilizing role in lower limb function [91].

5. Biomechanics and function

In open-chain movements, the adductors primarily produce hip adduction, with variable contributions to hip flexion, extension, and internal or external rotation depending on the muscle segment [50, 89].

In closed-chain conditions, such as single-leg stance or sport-specific maneuvers, they stabilize the pelvis, align the lower limb, and contribute to medial knee stability, limiting excessive valgus collapse [90]. These functions are essential during high-demand actions such as kicking, rapid changes of direction, and single-leg landings.

Appendices C. Quadriceps injuries

C.1 Anatomy and biomechanics

The quadriceps femoris is the largest muscle group of the anterior thigh and a key driver of human locomotion. Its anatomical complexity, spanning both the hip and knee joints through the rectus femoris, makes it crucial not only for knee extension but also for dynamic pelvic and gait stabilization [94].

1. Origins and insertions

The quadriceps femoris consists of four main muscles: rectus femoris, vastus lateralis, vastus medialis, and vastus intermedius [94]:

- Rectus femoris: It has two proximal heads. The superficial head arises from the anterior inferior iliac spine (AIIS), while the deep head originates from the acetabular rim. These fuse into a central aponeurotic tendon that runs through most of the muscle belly;
- Vastus lateralis: It originates from the greater trochanter and the lateral lip of the linea aspera. It inserts into the lateral patellar margin, contributing to the lateral retinaculum;
- Vastus medialis: It arises from the lower portion of the intertrochanteric line and the medial lip of the linea aspera. It inserts on the medial patellar margin, forming the medial retinaculum;
- Vastus intermedius: It originates from the anterior and lateral shaft of the femur and inserts deep into the quadriceps tendon.

All muscles converge into the quadriceps tendon, which envelopes the patella and continues distally as the patellar tendon, inserting on the tibial tuberosity [94].

2. Innervation and vascular supply

The quadriceps are innervated by the femoral nerve (L2–L4) [95, 96]. The anterior division supplies the sartorius, pectineus, and iliacus, while the posterior division innervates the quadriceps femoris group [96].

Blood supply comes primarily from the femoral artery and its deep branch, the profunda femoris, which gives rise to the medial and lateral circumflex arteries [97]. Lymphatic drainage occurs *via* the external iliac plexus, ultimately reaching the thoracic duct [98].

3. Relevant anatomical relationships

The quadriceps occupy the anterior thigh compartment, alongside the sartorius and pectineus [94]. They are closely related to the adductor canal, which serves as a conduit for the femoral artery and vein, the saphenous nerve, and the nerve to vastus medialis [94].

Functionally, the quadriceps interact with the patella. The vastus lateralis tends to pull the patella laterally, while the vastus medialis counterbalances this force, contributing to correct patellar tracking [94].

4. Anatomical variants

Reported variations include differences in the proximal origin of the rectus femoris heads, the length of its central tendon, and collateral vascularization from the circumflex branches [94].

5. Biomechanics and function

The quadriceps are the primary extensors of the knee and play a pivotal role in locomotion and dynamic stabilization [94, 99]:

- The rectus femoris is unique in crossing both the hip and knee joints. It contributes to hip flexion and stabilizes the pelvis during early gait.
- Quadriceps activation peaks during the early stance phase of walking and becomes more pronounced during climbing, sprinting, or jumping.
- The group plays a central role in eccentric control, decelerating the body during landings, braking, cutting, and downhill running.

The rectus femoris also helps control anterior pelvic translation during running and jumping through eccentric contraction [60]. A functional balance with the hamstrings is essential to maintain joint stability, reduce abnormal stress on the anterior cruciate ligament, and prevent knee injuries [100].

Author details

Loris Perticarini[1*], Luca Andriollo[1] and Francesco Benazzo[1,2]

1 Sports Traumatology Unit, Orthopedics and Traumatology, Fondazione Poliambulanza Istituto Ospedaliero, Brescia, Italy

2 IUSS Istituto Universitario di Studi Superiori, Pavia, Italy

*Address all correspondence to: loris.perticarini@gmail.com

References

[1] Palermi S, Vittadini F, Pedret C, Vecchiato M, Della Villa F, Corsini A, et al. From the field to the screen: A scoping review of video analysis as a tool for understanding thigh muscle-tendon injuries in football. Clinical Journal of Sport Medicine. 2022. DOI: 10.1097/JSM.0000000000001377

[2] Corsini A, Bisciotti A, Canonico R, Causarano A, Del Vescovo R, Gatto P, et al. Are football players more prone to muscle injury after COVID-19 infection? The "Italian injury study" during the serie a championship. International Journal of Environmental Research and Public Health. 2023;**20**(6):5182

[3] Hägglund M, Waldén M, Magnusson H, Kristenson K, Bengtsson H, Ekstrand J. Injuries affect team performance negatively in professional football: An 11-year follow-up of the UEFA champions league injury study. British Journal of Sports Medicine. 2013;**47**(12):738-742

[4] Ekstrand J, Hägglund M, Waldén M. Injury incidence and injury patterns in professional football: The UEFA injury study. British Journal of Sports Medicine. 2011;**45**(7):553-558

[5] Lundblad M, Waldén M, Magnusson H, Karlsson J, Ekstrand J. The UEFA injury study: 11-year data concerning 346 MCL injuries and time to return to play. British Journal of Sports Medicine. 2013;**47**(12):759-762

[6] Palmer B, McBride M, Jones G, Mayhew L. Injury trends in men's English professional football: An 11-year case series. Journal of Elite Sport Performance. 2023;**3**(1):1-8

[7] Ekstrand J, Waldén M, Hägglund M. Hamstring injuries have increased by 4% annually in men's professional football, since 2001: A 13-year longitudinal analysis of the UEFA elite club injury study. British Journal of Sports Medicine. 2016;**50**(12):731-737

[8] Garcia AG, Andrade R, Afonso J, Runco JL, Maestro A, Espregueira-Mendes J. Hamstrings injuries in football. Journal of Orthopaedics. 2022;**31**:72-77

[9] Serner A, Weir A, Tol JL, Thorborg K, Roemer F, Guermazi A, et al. Characteristics of acute groin injuries in the adductor muscles: A detailed MRI study in athletes. Scandinavian Journal of Medicine & Science in Sports. 2018;**28**(2):667-676

[10] Jokela A, Pasta G, Villa FD, Abrantes A, Kalogiannidis D, García-Romero-Pérez A, et al. Mechanisms of severe adductor longus injuries in professional soccer players: A systematic visual video analysis. The Orthopaedic Journal of Sports Medicine. 2025;**13**(2):23259671241309647

[11] Lempainen L, Mechó S, Valle X, Mazzoni S, Villalon J, Freschi M, et al. Management of anterior thigh injuries in soccer players: Practical guide. BMC Sports Science, Medicine and Rehabilitation. 2022;**14**:41

[12] Palermi S, Vittadini F, Pasta G, Zappia M, Corsini A, Pedret C, et al. The challenge of thigh tendon reinjuries: An expert opinion. Journal of Basic and Clinical Physiology and Pharmacology. 2024;**35**(6):335-345

[13] Palermi S, Vittadini F, Vecchiato M, Corsini A, Demeco A, Massa B, et al. Managing lower limb muscle reinjuries in athletes: From risk factors to

return-to-play strategies. Journal of Functional Morphology and Kinesiology. 2023;**8**(4):155

[14] Pollock N, James SLJ, Lee JC, Chakraverty R. British athletics muscle injury classification: A new grading system. British Journal of Sports Medicine. 2014;**48**(18):1347-1351

[15] Koulouris G, Connell D. Hamstring muscle complex: An imaging review. Radiographics: A Review Publication of the Radiological Society of North America, Inc. 2005;**25**(3):571-586

[16] Petersen J, Thorborg K, Nielsen MB, Skjødt T, Bolvig L, Bang N, et al. The diagnostic and prognostic value of ultrasonography in soccer players with acute hamstring injuries. The American Journal of Sports Medicine. 2014;**42**(2):399-404

[17] Balius R, Maestro A, Pedret C, Estruch A, Mota J, Rodríguez L, et al. Central aponeurosis tears of the rectus femoris: Practical sonographic prognosis. British Journal of Sports Medicine. 2009;**43**(11):818-824

[18] Isern-Kebschull J, Mechó S, Pruna R, Kassarjian A, Valle X, Yanguas X, et al. Sports-related lower limb muscle injuries: Pattern recognition approach and MRI review. Insights Into Imaging. 2020;**11**(1):108

[19] Heer ST, Callander JW, Kraeutler MJ, Mei-Dan O, Mulcahey MK. Hamstring injuries: Risk factors, treatment, and rehabilitation. The Journal of Bone and Joint Surgery. American Volume. 2019;**101**(9):843-853

[20] Bisciotti GN, Volpi P, Alberti G, Aprato A, Artina M, Auci A, et al. Italian consensus statement (2020) on return to play after lower limb muscle injury in football (soccer). BMJ Open Sport & Exercise Medicine. 2019;**5**(1):e000505

[21] Wangensteen A, Guermazi A, Tol JL, Roemer FW, Hamilton B, Alonso JM, et al. New MRI muscle classification systems and associations with return to sport after acute hamstring injuries: A prospective study. European Radiology. 2018;**28**(8):3532-3541

[22] Ishøi L, Krommes K, Husted RS, Juhl CB, Thorborg K. Diagnosis, prevention and treatment of common lower extremity muscle injuries in sport - grading the evidence: A statement paper commissioned by the Danish Society of Sports Physical Therapy (DSSF). British Journal of Sports Medicine. 2020;**54**(9):528-537

[23] Shamji R, James SLJ, Botchu R, Khurniawan KA, Bhogal G, Rushton A. Association of the British athletic muscle injury classification and anatomic location with return to full training and reinjury following hamstring injury in elite football. BMJ Open Sport & Exercise Medicine. 2021;**7**(2):e001010

[24] Valle X, Malliaropoulos N, Párraga Botero JD, Bikos G, Pruna R, Mónaco M, et al. Hamstring and other thigh injuries in children and young athletes. Scandinavian Journal of Medicine & Science in Sports. 2018;**28**(12):2630-2637

[25] Pollock N, Kelly S, Lee J, Stone B, Giakoumis M, Polglass G, et al. A 4-year study of hamstring injury outcomes in elite track and field using the British athletics rehabilitation approach. British Journal of Sports Medicine. 2022;**56**(5):257-263

[26] Mueller-Wohlfahrt HW, Haensel L, Mithoefer K, Ekstrand J, English B, McNally S, et al. Terminology and classification of muscle injuries in sport: The Munich consensus statement.

British Journal of Sports Medicine. 2013;**47**(6):342-350

[27] Ekstrand J, Askling C, Magnusson H, Mithoefer K. Return to play after thigh muscle injury in elite football players: Implementation and validation of the Munich muscle injury classification. British Journal of Sports Medicine. 2013;**47**(12):769-774

[28] Maffulli N, Oliva F, Frizziero A, Nanni G, Barazzuol M, Via AG, et al. ISMuLT guidelines for muscle injuries. Muscles, Ligaments and Tendons Journal. 2014;**3**(4):241-249

[29] Nanni G, Frizziero A, Di Miceli R, Vittadini F, Finotti P, Gamberini J, et al. Muscle injuries 2020 update of the I.S. Mu. L.T. classification. Muscles, Ligaments and Tendons Journal. 2020;**10**(4):562

[30] Mason DL, Dickens VA, Vail A. Rehabilitation for hamstring injuries. Cochrane Database of Systematic Reviews. 2012;**12**(12):CD004575

[31] Prior M, Guerin M, Grimmer K. An evidence-based approach to hamstring strain injury. Sports Health. 2009;**1**(2):154-164

[32] Sherry MA, Best TM. A comparison of 2 rehabilitation programs in the treatment of acute hamstring strains. The Journal of Orthopaedic and Sports Physical Therapy. 2004;**34**(3):116-125

[33] Petersen J, Hölmich P. Evidence based prevention of hamstring injuries in sport. British Journal of Sports Medicine. 2005;**39**(6):319-323

[34] Silvers-Granelli HJ, Cohen M, Espregueira-Mendes J, Mandelbaum B. Hamstring muscle injury in the athlete: State of the art. The Journal of ISAKOS. 2021;**6**(3):170-181

[35] Wood DG, Packham I, Trikha SP, Linklater J. Avulsion of the proximal hamstring origin. The Journal of Bone and Joint Surgery. American Volume. 2008;**90**(11):2365-2374

[36] Lempainen L, Sarimo J, Heikkilä J, Mattila K, Orava S. Surgical treatment of partial tears of the proximal origin of the hamstring muscles. British Journal of Sports Medicine. 2006;**40**(8):688-691

[37] Gronwald T, Klein C, Hoenig T, Pietzonka M, Bloch H, Edouard P, et al. Hamstring injury patterns in professional male football (soccer): A systematic video analysis of 52 cases. British Journal of Sports Medicine. 2022;**56**(3):165-171

[38] Heiderscheit BC, Sherry MA, Silder A, Chumanov ES, Thelen DG. Hamstring strain injuries: Recommendations for diagnosis, rehabilitation, and injury prevention. The Journal of Orthopaedic and Sports Physical Therapy. 2010;**40**(2):67-81

[39] Sarimo J, Lempainen L, Mattila K, Orava S. Complete proximal hamstring avulsions: A series of 41 patients with operative treatment. The American Journal of Sports Medicine. 2008;**36**(6):1110-1115

[40] Young IJ, van Riet RP, Bell SN. Surgical release for proximal hamstring syndrome. The American Journal of Sports Medicine. 2008;**36**(12):2372-2378

[41] Orchard JW, Chaker Jomaa M, Orchard JJ, Rae K, Hoffman DT, Reddin T, et al. Fifteen-week window for recurrent muscle strains in football: A prospective cohort of 3600 muscle strains over 23 years in professional Australian rules football. British Journal of Sports Medicine. 2020;**54**(18):1103-1107

[42] Piposar JR, Vinod AV, Olsen JR, Lacerte E, Miller SL. High-grade partial

and retracted (<2 cm) proximal hamstring ruptures: Nonsurgical treatment revisited. Orthopaedic Journal of Sports Medicine. 2017;**5**(2):2325967117692507

[43] Arner JW, McClincy MP, Bradley JP. Hamstring injuries in athletes: Evidence-based treatment. The Journal of the American Academy of Orthopaedic Surgeons. 2019;**27**(23):868-877

[44] Lempainen L, Banke IJ, Johansson K, Brucker PU, Sarimo J, Orava S, et al. Clinical principles in the management of hamstring injuries. Knee Surgery, Sports Traumatology, Arthroscopy. 2015;**23**(8):2449-2456

[45] Tyler TF, Silvers HJ, Gerhardt MB, Nicholas SJ. Groin injuries in sports medicine. Sports Health. 2010;**2**(3):231-236

[46] Farrell SG, Hatem M, Bharam S. Acute adductor muscle injury: A systematic review on diagnostic imaging, treatment, and prevention. The American Journal of Sports Medicine. 2023;**51**(13):3591-3603

[47] Lavoie-Gagne O, Mehta N, Patel S, Cohn MR, Forlenza E, Nwachukwu BU, et al. Adductor muscle injuries in UEFA soccer athletes: A matched-cohort analysis of injury rate, return to play, and player performance from 2000 to 2015. The Orthopaedic Journal of Sports Medicine. 2021;**9**(9):23259671211023098

[48] Whittaker JL, Small C, Maffey L, Emery CA. Risk factors for groin injury in sport: An updated systematic review. British Journal of Sports Medicine. 2015;**49**(12):803-809

[49] Quintana-Cepedal M, Vicente-Rodríguez G, Crespo I, Olmedillas H. Is hip adductor or abductor strength in healthy athletes associated with future groin pain? A systematic review and meta-analysis. British Journal of Sports Medicine. 2025;**59**(7):501-509

[50] Kai B, Lee KD, Andrews G, Wilkinson M, Forster BB. Puck to pubalgia: Imaging of groin pain in professional hockey players. Canadian Association of Radiologists Journal. 2010;**61**(2):74-79

[51] Serner A, Mosler AB, Tol JL, Bahr R, Weir A. Mechanisms of acute adductor longus injuries in male football players: A systematic visual video analysis. British Journal of Sports Medicine. 2019;**53**(3):158-164

[52] Bleakley CM, Glasgow P, MacAuley DC. PRICE needs updating, should we call the POLICE? British Journal of Sports Medicine. 2012;**46**(4):220-221

[53] Jensen J, Hölmich P, Bandholm T, Zebis MK, Andersen LL, Thorborg K. Eccentric strengthening effect of hip-adductor training with elastic bands in soccer players: A randomised controlled trial. British Journal of Sports Medicine. 2014;**48**(4):332-338

[54] Davis JA, Stringer MD, Woodley SJ. New insights into the proximal tendons of adductor longus, adductor brevis and gracilis. British Journal of Sports Medicine. 2012;**46**(12):871-876

[55] Serner A, Jakobsen MD, Andersen LL, Hölmich P, Sundstrup E, Thorborg K. EMG evaluation of hip adduction exercises for soccer players: Implications for exercise selection in prevention and treatment of groin injuries. British Journal of Sports Medicine. 2014;**48**(14):1108-1114

[56] Serner A, Weir A, Tol JL, Thorborg K, Lanzinger S, Otten R, et al. Return to sport after criteria-based rehabilitation of acute adductor injuries in male athletes: A prospective cohort

study. Orthopaedic Journal of Sports Medicine. 2020;**8**(1):2325967119897247

[57] Schlegel TF, Bushnell BD, Godfrey J, Boublik M. Success of nonoperative management of adductor longus tendon ruptures in national football league athletes. The American Journal of Sports Medicine. 2009;**37**(7):1394-1399

[58] Vogt S, Ansah P, Imhoff AB. Complete osseous avulsion of the adductor longus muscle: Acute repair with three fiberwire suture anchors. Archives of Orthopaedic and Trauma Surgery. 2007;**127**(8):613-615

[59] Schilders E, Dimitrakopoulou A, Cooke M, Bismil Q, Cooke C. Effectiveness of a selective partial adductor release for chronic adductor-related groin pain in professional athletes. The American Journal of Sports Medicine. 2013;**41**(3):603-607

[60] Mendiguchia J, Alentorn-Geli E, Idoate F, Myer GD. Rectus femoris muscle injuries in football: A clinically relevant review of mechanisms of injury, risk factors and preventive strategies. British Journal of Sports Medicine. 2013;**47**(6):359-366

[61] Cloke D, Moore O, Shab T, Rushton S, Shirley MDF, Deehan DJ. Thigh muscle injuries in youth soccer: Predictors of recovery. The American Journal of Sports Medicine. 2012;**40**(2):433-439

[62] Kassarjian A, Rodrigo RM, Santisteban JM. Current concepts in MRI of rectus femoris musculotendinous (myotendinous) and myofascial injuries in elite athletes. European Journal of Radiology. 2012;**81**(12):3763-3771

[63] Pietsch S, Pizzari T. Risk factors for quadriceps muscle strain injuries in sport: A systematic review. The Journal of Orthopaedic and Sports Physical Therapy. 2022;**52**(6):389-400

[64] Fousekis K, Tsepis E, Poulmedis P, Athanasopoulos S, Vagenas G. Intrinsic risk factors of non-contact quadriceps and hamstring strains in soccer: A prospective study of 100 professional players. British Journal of Sports Medicine. 2011;**45**(9):709-714

[65] Kary JM. Diagnosis and management of quadriceps strains and contusions. Current Reviews in Musculoskeletal Medicine. 2010;**3**(1-4):26-31

[66] Ackermann PW, Renström P. Tendinopathy in sport. Sports Health. 2012;**4**(3):193-201

[67] Saragaglia D, Pison A, Rubens-Duval B. Acute and old ruptures of the extensor apparatus of the knee in adults (excluding knee replacement). Orthopaedics & Traumatology: Surgery & Research. 2013;**99**(1 Suppl):S67-S76

[68] Hak DJ, Sanchez A, Trobisch P. Quadriceps tendon injuries. Orthopedics. 2010;**33**(1):40-46

[69] Lempainen L, Kosola J, Niemi P, Orava S, Pruna R. Complete midsubstance rectus femoris ruptures: A series of 27 athletes treated operatively. Muscle Ligaments Tendons Journal. 2019;**08**(02):276

[70] Lempainen L, Kosola J, Pruna R, Puigdellivol J, Ranne J, Orava S. Operative treatment of proximal rectus femoris injuries in professional soccer players: A series of 19 cases. Orthopaedic Journal of Sports Medicine. 2018;**6**(10):2325967118798827

[71] Prisk V, Huard J. Muscle injuries and repair: The role of prostaglandins and inflammation. Histology and Histopathology. 2003;**18**(4):1243-1256

[72] Pieters D, Wezenbeek E, Schuermans J, Witvrouw E. Return to

play after a hamstring strain injury: It is time to consider natural healing. Sports Medicine (Auckland, N.Z.). 2021;**51**(10):2067-2077

[73] Plesser S, Keilani M, Vekszler G, Hasenoehrl T, Palma S, Reschl M, et al. Clinical outcomes after treatment of quadriceps tendon ruptures show equal results independent of suture anchor or transosseus repair technique used - a pilot study. PLoS One. 2018;**13**(3):e0194376

[74] Jokela A, Stenroos A, Kosola J, Valle X, Lempainen L. A systematic review of surgical intervention in the treatment of hamstring tendon ruptures: Current evidence on the impact on patient outcomes. Annals of Medicine. 2022;**54**(1):978-988

[75] Allahabadi S, Salazar LM, Obioha OA, Fenn TW, Chahla J, Nho SJ. Hamstring injuries: A current concepts review: Evaluation, nonoperative treatment, and surgical decision making. The American Journal of Sports Medicine. 2024;**52**(3):832-844

[76] Rodgers CD, Raja A. Anatomy, Bony Pelvis and Lower Limb, Hamstring Muscle. Treasure Island (FL): StatPearls Publishing; 2025. Disponibile su: http://www.ncbi.nlm.nih.gov/books/NBK546688/ [Accessed: agosto 17, 2025]

[77] Tomaszewski KA, Henry BM, Vikse J, Pękala P, Roy J, Svensen M, et al. Variations in the origin of the deep femoral artery: A meta-analysis. Clinical Anatomy N Y N. 2017;**30**(1):106-113

[78] Choy KW, Kogilavani S, Norshalizah M, Rani S, Aspalilah A, Hamzi H, et al. Topographical anatomy of the profunda femoris artery and the femoral nerve: Normal and abnormal relationships. La Clinica Terapeutica. 2013;**164**(1):17-19

[79] Greenwood K, N ZR v K, Hohmann E. Defining the popliteal fossa by bony landmarks and mapping of the courses of the neurovascular structures for application in popliteal fossa surgery. Anatomy & Cell Biology. 2021;**54**(1):10-17

[80] Chakravarthi K. Unusual unilateral multiple muscular variations of back of thigh. The Annals of Medical and Health Sciences Research. 2013;**3**(Suppl 1):S1-S2

[81] Sussmann AR. Congenital bilateral absence of the semimembranosus muscles. Skeletal Radiology. 2019;**48**(10):1651-1655

[82] Park JH, Park KR, Yang J, Park GH, Cho J. Unusual variant of distal biceps femoris muscle associated with common peroneal entrapment neuropathy: A cadaveric case report. Medicine (Baltimore). 2018;**97**(38):e12274

[83] Woodley SJ, Mercer SR. Hamstring muscles: Architecture and innervation. Cells, Tissues, Organs. 2005;**179**(3):125-141

[84] Woods C, Hawkins RD, Maltby S, Hulse M, Thomas A, Hodson A, et al. The football association medical research programme: An audit of injuries in professional football--analysis of hamstring injuries. British Journal of Sports Medicine. 2004;**38**(1):36-41

[85] Gabbe BJ, Finch CF, Bennell KL, Wajswelner H. Risk factors for hamstring injuries in community level Australian football. British Journal of Sports Medicine. 2005;**39**(2):106-110

[86] Tubbs RS, Griessenauer CJ, Marshall T, Dennison CP, Shoja MM, Loukas M, et al. The adductor minimus muscle revisited. Surgical and Radiologic Anatomy SRA. 2011;**33**(5):429-432

[87] Launico MV, Sinkler MA, Nallamothu SV. Anatomy, Bony Pelvis and Lower Limb: Femoral Muscles. Treasure Island (FL): StatPearls Publishing; 2025. Disponibile su: http://www.ncbi.nlm.nih.gov/books/NBK500008/ [Accessed: agosto 16, 2025]

[88] Takizawa M, Suzuki D, Ito H, Fujimiya M, Uchiyama E. Why adductor magnus muscle is large: The function based on muscle morphology in cadavers. Scandinavian Journal of Medicine & Science in Sports. 2014;**24**(1):197-203

[89] Benn ML, Pizzari T, Rath L, Tucker K, Semciw AI. Adductor magnus: An EMG investigation into proximal and distal portions and direction specific action. Clinical Anatomy N Y N. 2018;**31**(4):535-543

[90] Jeno SH, Launico MV, Schindler GS. Anatomy, Bony Pelvis and Lower Limb: Thigh Adductor Magnus Muscle. Treasure Island (FL): StatPearls Publishing; 2025. Disponibile su: http://www.ncbi.nlm.nih.gov/books/NBK534842/ [Accessed: agosto 17, 2025]

[91] Takizawa M, Suzuki D, Ito H, Fujimiya M, Uchiyama E. The adductor part of the adductor magnus is innervated by both obturator and sciatic nerves. Clinical Anatomy N Y N. 2014;**27**(5):778-782

[92] Schilders E, Bharam S, Golan E, Dimitrakopoulou A, Mitchell A, Spaepen M, et al. The pyramidalis-anterior pubic ligament-adductor longus complex (PLAC) and its role with adductor injuries: A new anatomical concept. Knee Surgery, Sports Traumatology, Arthroscopy. 2017;**25**(12):3969-3977

[93] Tubbs RS, Loukas M, Shoja MM, Apaydin N, Oakes WJ, Salter EG. Anatomy and potential clinical significance of the vastoadductor membrane. Surgical and Radiologic Anatomy SRA. 2007;**29**(7):569-573

[94] Khan A, Arain A. Anatomy, Bony Pelvis and Lower Limb: Anterior Thigh Muscles. Treasure Island (FL): StatPearls Publishing; 2025. Disponibile su: http://www.ncbi.nlm.nih.gov/books/NBK538425/ [Accessed: agosto 17, 2025]

[95] Grob K, Manestar M, Filgueira L, Ackland T, Gilbey H, Kuster MS. New insight in the architecture of the quadriceps tendon. Journal of Experimental Orthopaedics. 2016;**3**(1):32

[96] Page BJ, Mrowczynski OD, Payne RA, Tilden SE, Lopez H, Rizk E, et al. The relative location of the major femoral nerve motor branches in the thigh. Cureus; 2019;**11**(1):e3882

[97] Tomaszewski KA, Vikse J, Henry BM, Roy J, Pękala PA, Svensen M, et al. The variable origin of the lateral circumflex femoral artery: A meta-analysis and proposal for a new classification system. Folia Morphologica. 2017;**76**(2):157-167

[98] Ramage JL, Varacallo MA. Anatomy, Bony Pelvis and Lower Limb: Medial Thigh Muscles. Treasure Island (FL): StatPearls Publishing; 2025. Disponibile su: http://www.ncbi.nlm.nih.gov/books/NBK534775/ [Accessed: agosto 17, 2025]

[99] Sasaki K, Neptune RR. Individual muscle contributions to the axial knee joint contact force during normal walking. Journal of Biomechanics. 2010;**43**(14):2780-2784

[100] Lehr ME, Plisky PJ, Butler RJ, Fink ML, Kiesel KB, Underwood FB. Field-expedient screening and injury risk algorithm categories as predictors of noncontact lower extremity injury. Scandinavian Journal of Medicine & Science in Sports. 2013;**23**(4):e225-e232

Chapter 5

Achilles Tendon Injury Management

Meshal Alhadhoud

Abstract

Achilles tendon injuries, encompassing acute ruptures, represent a significant cause of morbidity, particularly in active individuals. Effective management requires an accurate diagnosis, typically achieved through clinical assessment supplemented by ultrasound or MRI, to differentiate between rupture and other conditions. Treatment strategies are tailored to the type of injury, factors related to the patient (such as age and activity level), and tear characteristics. For acute ruptures, management involves a critical choice between a non-operative functional rehabilitation protocol and operative repair. Nonoperative protocols utilize early functional bracing with controlled, progressive ankle mobilization, demonstrating comparable outcomes to surgery in many patients while avoiding surgical risks. Surgical intervention (open or minimally invasive (closed percutaneous or semi-open) repair) is often preferred for younger, highly active individuals, complete tears, or delayed presentations, although it carries risks of infection and wound complications. Rehabilitation is paramount across all injury types, emphasizing structured, graded loading to restore tendon capacity, strength, and function, followed by sport-specific retraining. Prevention strategies emphasize the importance of load monitoring, maintaining calf strength, and addressing biomechanical risk factors. Future directions include optimizing biological augmentation and refining accelerated rehabilitation protocols. A multidisciplinary, evidence-based approach ensures optimal functional recovery and minimizes the risk of re-rupture.

Keywords: Achilles tendon rupture, Achilles tendinopathy, functional rehabilitation, surgical repair, heavy slow resistance training, eccentric exercise, tendon loading

1. Introduction

Acute Achilles tendon rupture (ATR) is common in recreational athletics in the younger age group, and more than two-thirds are sport activity-related [1, 2]. The ATR incidence is varying from different countries, reported from 1.8 to 51.3 per 100,000 person-years, and the trend is increasing [3].

The literature comprises multiple and conflicting data regarding the pathophysiology and treatment approaches for Achilles tendon rupture. There are over 800 articles in the literature, and it is impractical to cite and discuss all the evidence of management methodology. The purpose of this chapter is to present a highly evidence-based clinical evaluation and management of Achilles tendon rupture.

IntechOpen

The main question raised for any orthopedic surgeon treating Achilles tendon rupture is to manage this injury with operative or non-operative management [4]. Each management has its risks and benefits. Non-operative management has a lower complication rate compared with operative management [4]. Wound problems are more with operative management, and the non-operative management has a higher rate of re-rupture. Another issue is about rehabilitation – whether to use a functional protocol or a traditional casting with a non-weight-bearing protocol. Harrington et al. found in the review article the lowest re-rupture rate achieved with the use of a functional rehabilitation protocol involving protected weight-bearing. However, these results are consistent with Ochen et al., who compared a functional rehabilitation protocol with a traditional protocol and found re-rupture rates of 3.9 and 9 to 13%, respectively [4, 5].

2. Anatomy

The Achilles tendon, named after the invincible Greek Warrior Achilles, is the largest in the body. It is formed by the gastrocnemius and soleus muscles, which spiral toward its insertion on the calcaneus [1]. The tendon lacks a genuine synovial sheath; it consists of paratenon with visceral and parietal layers, allowing about 1.5 cm of glide [1]. The main blood supply originates from the musculotendinous junction, osseous insertion, and mesotenal vessels, with a vascular watershed area located 2–6 cm proximal to the insertion, predisposing this zone to injury [1].

The triceps surae (gastrocnemius-soleus-complex) traverses the ankle and knee joint and distally consolidates to the Achilles tendon. The triceps surae is innervated by the tibial nerve [6]. The origin of the gastrocnemius is from the posterior aspect of the femoral condyle, and it is a plantar flexor of the ankle with the knee in extension. However, the soleus originates from the posterior aspect of the tibia, fibula, and interosseous membrane, and it is an effective plantar flexor of the ankle with the knee in flexion [7]. The Achilles tendon insertion is on the calcaneus tuberosity with a big surface area on the posterosuperior aspect [8]. There are two bursae at the Achilles tendon insertion: the retrocalcaneal bursa and the Achilles tendon bursa, located between the Achilles tendon and the calcaneus and the skin and tendon, respectively [9]. The anatomy of the Achilles tendon exposes it to multiple factors that can lead to wound complications. A thin layer of skin covers it and has a tenuous blood supply [10]. Understanding the anatomy of the Achilles tendon, including vascular mapping, helps us avoid the associated complications post-surgery. Horacio et al. described the arterial blood supply to the Achilles tendon. The medial region has three to four small branches that come from the posterior tibial artery [10]. In contrast, the lateral region is supplied by three to four branches that come from the peroneal artery or its recurrent branch [10]. Therefore, the recommendation is to make a medical incision about 1 cm medial to the edge of the Achilles tendon and preserve the paratenon with minimized subcutaneous dissection [10].

3. Aetiology

The gastrocnemius-soleus-Achilles complex spans three joints and contributes to knee flexion, ankle plantar flexion, and subtalar supination. The rotational stress from the subtalar and knee movements contributes to tendon loading [1]. During running, forces on the tendon can reach up to ten times the body weight [1]. Achilles tendon rupture may result from underlying pathology, such as paratenonitis or tendinosis, in which the patient experiences prodromal symptoms, including tendon burning pain after activity or painless palpable nodules [1].

The disruption can occur anywhere along the length of the Achilles tendon, but the most common area of disruption is 2 to 6 cm proximal to the calcaneus insertion [11].

The mechanism of injury is either direct or indirect. The history of direct trauma is uncommon. However, it could include a direct blow to the posterior ankle, a crush injury, or a laceration.

The indirect mechanism of injury is the most reported type and includes mechanical stress and intratendinous pathology. There are three main mechanisms of indirect injury, including overloading, which results in tendon failure, the weight-bearing foot while the knee in extension, and forceful dorsiflexion on the planter-flexed ankle [2]. The Achilles tendon is a viscoelastic material; if the modulus of elasticity increases, the tendon becomes stiffer, and with a rapid loading process, it becomes more prone to rupture [7].

A deficit in the biomechanical alignment of the lower limb, such as hyperpronation, cavus foot, and forefoot varus, increases the risk of injury, particularly poorly absorbed shock, and stresses the lateral aspect of the tendon [1]. Tendon overuse injury and age have a positive predictive value in decreasing the blood supply, which can result in tendon rupture [1]. Inappropriate training, such as a sudden increase in intensity, excessive training, or running on a hard surface while wearing insufficient heel height and a rigid sole, can lead to injury [1]. The Achilles tendon comprises tenocytes embedded in an extracellular matrix of collagen, elastin, and glycoproteins. Aging results in decreased cell density, collagen fibril diameter, and fiber waviness, which increase injury susceptibility [1].

According to the recent systematic review of the risk factors of Achilles tendon rupture, there was low to very low evidence for medication such as steroids, quinolones, and oral bisphosphonates, and low to very low evidence for chronic tenon inflammation and Achilles tendinopathies [12].

4. Clinical signs

Rupture of the tendon is accompanied by sharp pain and a palpable tendon defect, and inability of the patient to do a single heel rise [1]. Simmonds-Thompson test is positive but may be masked by the presence of accessory flexors [1].

5. Diagnostic investigation

Diagnostics usually complements the history and physical examination (with special tests, like Simmonds-Thompson's, Matles' etc.); it is rarely indicated for special diagnostic studies [13–16]. Plan ankle radiographic AP and lateral views may be performed to show any associated pathology of the Achilles tendon, like tendon calcification or associated fracture of the calcaneus or any tarsal bone. However, plain radiography may show soft tissue swelling and changes in Kager's triangle, indicating an Achilles tendon rupture [13].

Ultrasonography is another modality that can be used in radiographic examination, and it is a valuable tool in detecting any pathological conditions affecting the Achilles tendon [17]. Ultrasonography has a high specificity, ranging from 83 to 100%, and a sensitivity range of 72 to 94% [18].

MRI is very sensitive in detecting intratendinous lesions with a positive predictive value of 94% [19]. It's considered a comprehensive diagnostic tool for Achilles tendon injuries. It gives more details on incomplete ruptures, tendon fatty infiltration, and degeneration. The significant limitations of MRI are cost, inconvenience for patients with claustrophobia, and oversensitivity, which may show areas of change that are not clinically relevant [19].

6. Management of Achilles tendon rupture

6.1 Functional rehabilitation

Historically, the treatment of ATR was non-operative in the 1800s and 1900s. In the early 1920s, the surgical treatment of Achilles tendon rupture was first introduced and gradually increased [20]. In 1981, Nistor published a prospective, randomized study advocating that there is no difference in surgical and nonsurgical treatment of Achilles tendon rupture. Since then, nonsurgical treatment has become gradually more popular [21], until later dynamometric and clinical studies showed superior functional results in operative treatment [22].

An accelerated functional rehabilitation program has changed the concept of increased re-rupture rates with conservative treatment of Achilles tendon rupture [3]. A meta-analysis of 826 patients comparing operative and non-operative groups who underwent a functional rehabilitation protocol found that early range of motion had an equal re-rupture rate compared to the operative group (risk difference = 1.7%, P = 0.45) [4]. There are many options for immobilization and orthosis use: primarily, custom-made splints, or semi-rigid orthoses [3]. However, the rigid protocol to use these orthotics along with a functional rehabilitation protocol to achieve a plantar flexion of the foot for about 25 to 30 degrees, and after 3 to 4 weeks in a neutral position [3].

The main inclusion criteria for non-operative treatment are that the patient has had non or minimal weight-bearing and diagnosed within 2 days [23]. The patient undergoes immobilization in the maximum passive plantar flexion position for 2 weeks [23]. At the 2-week follow-up visit, the patient was fitted with a specific Achilles walking boot featuring 40-degree heel lifts and initiated the Glazbrook/Rubinger Achilles Protocol for Nonoperative Treatment (GAPNOT) [23]. The key feature is that the patient starts weight bearing 25% of his weight each week till the patient reaches a full weight bearing at week 6 and the start to remove the one shoe lift daily starting from week 6 and weaning of the boot walker which needs a compliance from the patient to increase the successful outcome [23]. At this time, the patient is instructed not to pass 90 degrees of ankle dorsiflexion, especially during the 2- to 8-week stage. A conventional physiotherapy modality and active heel rise accompanied by electric muscle stimulation in the sitting position are performed [23]. Between weeks 8 and 12, the patient starts active plantarflexion and strengthening exercises; however, no activities are performed that dorsiflex the ankle past 90 degrees. At this stage, the patient can use a stationary bicycle with minimal resistance and perform close kinetic chain exercises to strengthen the kinetic chain, as well as double heel rises [23]. From weeks 12 to 16, it is a critical stage where the re-rupture and elongation of the tendon may occur because the patient returns to their normal activity level. Therefore, educating the patient is essential at this stage, and patient compliance in attending physiotherapy is substantial [23]. At the 4- to 6-month stage, the patient is performing his strengthening exercises, and there is a periodic check with physiotherapy to ensure no tendon elongation has occurred. At this stage, the patient should be able to do a single heel rise. After 6 months, the patient should return to his sports activities but should be instructed to avoid any contact sports. Between 9 and 12 months, the patient should return for full sports activity [23].

During this period, the surgeon should follow-up with the patient at 2, 6, 12, 26, and 52 weeks. During these visits, the surgeon will assess the healing process and take a clear history and physical examination, look for pain, swelling, and ecchymosis, and assess the filling gap [23]. Also, the surgeon will evaluate the length of the Achilles tendon and ankle range of motion by passive dorsiflexion with the knee in extension and compare it with the contralateral side. Moreover, the surgeon will continue educating the patients and encourage them to adhere to the physiotherapy protocol [23].

6.1.1 Accelerated functional rehabilitation protocol

See **Table 1**.

0–2 weeks	• Below-knee plaster cast with the ankle held in planter flexion; non-weight bearing using crutches.

2–4 weeks	• Boot walking with 40-degree or 30-degree planter-flexed heel lift
	• Protected weight bearing with crutches:
	  o Weeks 2–3—25
	  o Weeks 3–4—50%
	  o Weeks 4–5—75%
	  o Weeks 5–6—100%
	• Start active ROM dorsiflexion and plantarflexion (to neutral), while inversion, eversion under neutral
	• Use different modalities to reduce swelling
	• Muscle stimulation using electrical muscle stimulation machines while the patient is seated
	• Patients visit the physiotherapy clinic 2–3 times a week to assess the swelling and pain
	• Involve the upper joints knee and hip in the exercise without involvement of the ankle
	• Fitness and cardio workout should not start until 3–4 weeks and should be non-weight-bearing
	• Hydrotherapy will help with limitation of motion
	• Always keep pain as a guide to decrease the exercise intensity.

4–6 weeks	• Continuation weight bearing as tolerated • Continue 2–4-week protocol • Progress with electrical muscle stimulation with no resistance • The ankle should not pass neutral • Continue with physiotherapy 2–3 times/wk. • Patient can do fitness and cardio exercise with boot walker on.

6–8 weeks	• Continue physiotherapy two times per week • Continue swelling decreasing modalities • Progress with electrical muscle stimulation with no resistance • The ankle should not pass neutral • Start to remove one heel lift daily depends on patient tolerance and Achilles length • Full weight-bearing with boot walker • Start open and close chain kinetic functional exercises • Do not go past the neutral ankle position • Started gait training with full weight-bearing • Exercise fitness and cardio with full weight-bearing, for example, biking • Hydrotherapy
8–12 weeks	Patient education in this stage is mandatory. The patient should understand that the tendon is still at risk of reinjured. The patient should take care with activity of daily living and exercise any sudden loading will result in re-rupture. • Wean off the boot and wear an Achilles compression ankle brace with the shoes • Wean off crutches and cane gradually • Progress to strengthen and proprioception exercise add balance board but block it at dorsiflexion to prevent pass neutral • Start elliptical training or stationary bicycle • Add calf stretches in standing do not allow the ankle to go past the neutral position. • Add double-heel raises and progress to single-heel raises when tolerated. Do not allow the ankle to go past the neutral position. • Continue physiotherapy 1–2 times per week.
12–16weeks	• Continue ROM, strength, and proprioception exercises • Retrain strength, power, and endurance Patient education is important; still Achilles tendon is vulnerable. Prevention of any heavy exercise put the tendon on stress.
16+ weeks	• Increase the exercise intensity, for example, jogging, weight training, and skipping.
6–9 months	• If the patient regains 80% of strength can involve in sporting activity that involved sprinting, cutting, and jumping.
12 months	• 100% regaining of the strength; the patient can return to the same level of activity pre-injury with medical team direction.

Table 1.
Glazebrook/Rubinger Achilles protocol for nonoperative treatment (GAPNOT) [23].

6.2 Operative treatment

Operative treatment consists of open surgical and minimally invasive (whether closed percutaneous or minimally open (MIO), with costly devices) repair [3, 24, 25].

Recent evidence has shown same functional outcomes and re-rupture rates between operative and non-operative groups with an accelerated functional rehabilitation protocol, including early weight-bearing and range of motion of the ankle [22, 24]. On the contrary, with immobilization and restricted ankle range of motion, this could increase the chance of re-rupture [22, 24].

A systematic review and meta-analysis including eight randomized control trails involving 762 patients shows re-rupture rate is 3.7% in operative group and 9.8% in non-operative group, and the pooled results were significantly lower in the operative group than nonoperative [24].

In a multicenter randomized control trail comparing a non-operative treatment, open repair, and minimal invasive (MIO) surgery, this study includes 554 patients. The mean change in Achilles re-rupture score was −17.0 points in the nonoperative group, −16.0 points in the open repair group, and – 14.7 points in the minimally invasive group. This shows no evidence of difference between the groups [25].

A recent comparative study includes 434 patients comparing Percutaneous Achillis Repair System (PARS) and Midsubstance Speedbridge Impant System (MSB). There is no significance difference in a patient functional outcome and postoperative complication [26].

A systematic review and meta-analysis focused on different types of surgical approach combining them with traditional standard rehabilitation and functional accelerated rehabilitation protocol include 38 randomized controlled trials involving 2480 patients shows minimal invasive repair has low risk of complication, and accelerated functional rehabilitation protocol superior to traditional standard rehabilitation, however, combination of minimal invasive repair and accelerated functional rehabilitation protocol has the best therapeutic protocol [27].

Comparing the complication rate between minimal invasive and open repair was a debatable subject. However, recent evidence reveals that both techniques have a comparable complication rate. However, patient factors, such as increased BMI and delayed presentation, contribute to a slight increase in complications in the open repair group [28].

Choosing between operative and non-operative treatment is a shared decision-making process between the surgeon and the patient. The surgeon should continually educate the patient about the two treatment modalities and explain the risks and benefits of each to them and then let the patient choose the most suitable option. Unless the patient has specific factors that the surgeon thinks would be better suited for either surgical or nonsurgical treatment, the patient should be allowed to make the decision [29, 30].

7. Conclusions

The accuracy of history taking and physical examination, combined with the addition of radiological examination, is the most helpful factor for accurate diagnosis in the initial presentation. The decision-making for treatment depends on multiple factors. However, the decision for non-surgical treatment is still a good option if the patient fits the criteria and surgical treatment has versatile options from MIS to open technique. Overall, the decision-making should be shared with the patient. A functional rehabilitation protocol with early weight-bearing proved to have significantly better functional outcomes.

Acknowledgements

The author thanks his colleagues at Al-Adan Hospital for their stimulating discussions and to his wife, Hessah, for her unwavering support."

Conflict of interest

The author declares no conflict of interest.

Author details

Meshal Alhadhoud
Ministry of Health, Al-Adan Hospital, Hadiya, Kuwait

*Address all correspondence to: maalhadhoud@gmail.com

References

[1] Saltzman CL, Tearse DS. Achilles tendon injuries. The Journal of the American Academy of Orthopaedic Surgeons. 1998;**6**(5):316-325

[2] Čretnik A, Košir R. Incidence of Achilles tendon rupture: 25-year regional analysis with a focus on bilateral ruptures. Journal of International Medical Research. 2023;**51**(11):1-12

[3] Čretnik A. In: Nikolopoulos DD, Safos GK, editors. Functional Rehabilitation after Achilles Tendon Rupture. England: IntechOpen; 2023. p. 365. DOI: 10.5772/intechopen.111568

[4] Harrington TL, Breedlove GJ, Sharpe JJ. Systematic review of nonoperative functional protocols for acute Achilles ruptures utilizing a formal rehabilitation protocol showing lowest rerupture rates. Foot and Ankle Specialist. 2020;**13**:508-515

[5] Ochen Y, Beks RB, Van Heijl M, Hietbrink F, Leenen LPH, Van Der Velde D, et al. Operative treatment versus nonoperative treatment of Achilles tendon ruptures: Systematic review and meta-analysis. BMJ. 2019;**364**:k5120

[6] Lemm M, Blake RL, Colson JP, Ferguson H, Achilles peritendinitis. A literature review with case report. Journal of the American Podiatric Medical Association. 1992;**82**(9): 482-490

[7] DeMaio M, Paine R, Drez DJJ. Achilles tendonitis. Orthopedics. 1995;**18**(2):195-204

[8] Chao W, Deland JT, Bates JE, Kenneally SM. Achilles tendon insertion: An in vitro anatomic study. Foot & Ankle International. 1997;**18**(2):81-84

[9] Fuglsang F, Torup D. Bursitis retrocalcanearis. Acta Orthopaedica Scandinavica. 1961;**30**:315-323

[10] Yepes H, Tang M, Geddes C, Glazebrook M, Morris SF, Stanish WD. Digital vascular mapping of the integument about the Achilles tendon. The Journal of Bone and Joint Surgery. American Volume. 2010;**92**(5):1215-1220

[11] Liu S, Ma L. Minimally invasive internal splinting technique for acute closed Achilles tendon rupture. Journal of Orthopaedic Surgery and Research. 2025;**20**:116

[12] Xergia SA, Tsarbou C, Liveris NI, Hadjithoma M, Tzanetakou IP. Risk factors for Achilles tendon rupture: An updated systematic review. Physician and Sportsmedicine. 2023;**51**(6):506-516

[13] Hattrup SJ, Johnson KA. A review of ruptures of the Achilles tendon. Foot & Ankle. 1985;**6**(1):34-38

[14] Simmonds FA. The diagnosis of the ruptured Achilles tendon. The Practitioner. 1957;**179**(1069):56-58

[15] Thompson TC. A test for rupture of the tendo achillis. Acta Orthopaedica Scandinavica. 1962;**32**:461-465

[16] Maffulli N. The clinical diagnosis of subcutaneous tear of the Achilles tendon. A prospective study in 174 patients. The American Journal of Sports Medicine [Internet]. 1998;**26**(2):266-270. Available from: http://www.ncbi.nlm.nih.gov/pubmed/9548122

[17] Lehtinen A, Peltokallio P, Taavitsainen M. Sonography of Achilles tendon correlated to operative findings. Annales Chirurgiae et Gynaecologiae. 1994;**83**(4):322-327

[18] Kälebo P, Allenmark C, Peterson L, Swärd L. Diagnostic value of ultrasonography in partial ruptures of the Achilles tendon. The American Journal of Sports Medicine. 1992;**20**(4):378-381

[19] Panageas E, Greenberg S, Franklin PD, Carter AP, Bloom D. Magnetic resonance imaging of pathologic conditions of the Achilles tendon. Orthopaedic Review. 1990;**19**(11):975-980

[20] Fierro NL, Sallis RE. Achilles tendon rupture. Is casting enough? Postgraduate Medicine. 1995;**98**(3):145-152

[21] Nistor L. Surgical and non-surgical treatment of Achilles tendon rupture. A prospective randomized study. The Journal of Bone and Joint Surgery. American Volume. 1981;**63**(3): 394-399

[22] Soroceanu A, Sidhwa F, Aarabi S, Kaufman A, Glazebrook M. Surgical versus nonsurgical treatment of acute Achilles tendon rupture: A meta-analysis of randomized trials. The Journal of Bone and Joint Surgery. American Volume. 2012;**94**(23):2136-2143

[23] Glazebrook M, Rubinger D. Functional rehabilitation for nonsurgical treatment of acute Achilles tendon rupture. Foot and Ankle Clinics [Internet]. 2019;**24**(3):387-398. DOI: 10.1016/j.fcl.2019.05.001

[24] Deng S, Sun Z, Zhang C, Chen G, Li J. Surgical treatment versus conservative management for acute Achilles tendon rupture: A systematic review and meta-analysis of randomized controlled trials. Journal of Foot and Ankle Surgery [Internet]. 2017;**56**(6):1236-1243. DOI: 10.1053/j.jfas.2017.05.036

[25] Myhrvold SB, Brouwer EF, Andresen TKM, Rydevik K, Amundsen M, Grün W, et al. Nonoperative or surgical treatment of Acute Achilles' tendon rupture. New England Journal of Medicine. 2022;**386**(15):1409-1420

[26] Peabody JJ, Hadley SM, Bergman R, Westvold SJ, Olamigoke FO, Chang S, et al. Functional outcomes following minimally invasive Achilles rupture repair: A retrospective comparative study of PARS and midsubstance speedbridge techniques. Journal of Orthopaedic Surgery and Research. 2025;**20**:390

[27] Shi F, Wu S, Cai W, Zhao Y. Multiple comparisons of the efficacy and safety for six treatments in acute Achilles tendon rupture patients: A systematic review and network meta-analysis. Foot and Ankle Surgery. 2021;**27**:468-479

[28] Hendriks JRH, Sharma S, Peiffer M, de Groot TM, Waryasz G, Kerkhoffs GMMJ, et al. Postoperative complications after acute Achilles tendon rupture repair: A survival analysis of minimally invasive vs open techniques. Foot & Ankle International. 2025;**46**(7):707-714

[29] King CM, Vartivarian M. Achilles tendon rupture repair: Simple to complex. Clinics in Podiatric Medicine and Surgery. 2023;**40**(1):75-96

[30] Alrabaa RG, Freibott C, Vosseller JT. Patient perception of Achilles tendon rupture treatment. Injury. 2020;**51**(11):2710-2716

Chapter 6

A Review of Advances in Achilles Tendon Repair: Balancing Biomechanics and Biology

Sedeek M. Mosaid, Ashok Marudanayagam, Rizwan Shahid and Mohamed Elnemr

Abstract

This chapter explores the current innovations and challenges in tendon repair surgery, focusing on the delicate balance between mechanical stability and biological healing. The chapter critically discusses biomechanical principles of tendon repair, diverse suturing techniques, and the importance of timing in rehabilitation. It also addresses the role of biological augmentation techniques in enhancing tendon healing. Surgical tips and outcome-based comparisons have been included to provide surgeons with a comprehensive, practical perspective. Special attention is given to common clinical dilemmas such as managing and repairing degenerative tendons, delayed presentation, and management in elderly or active patients.

Keywords: tendon repair, mini-invasive techniques, tendon healing, biomechanics, biological augmentation, rehabilitation

1. Introduction

The Achilles tendon (AT) is the largest tendon in the lower limb and the most commonly injured tendon. It is used in activities like running and jumping, so it is prone to overuse injuries during sports and other physical activities [1].

Spontaneous rupture is reported to be increasing, probably due to demographic changes such as a growing elderly population and increased recreational activity among middle-aged individuals [2].

Although most AT ruptures occur during athletic activities, intrinsic structural, biochemical and biomechanical changes may also play a role. Injuries to the AT are often the result of repeated minor traumatic events rather than a single major incident [1, 2].

Other contributors to AT injury are chronic inflammation, degenerative changes in the tendon, and systemic conditions like diabetes mellitus, which can affect tissue quality. For example, diabetes can impair the overall health of the tendon and increase the risk of injury [1].

There is ongoing debate about the best treatment approach, as outcomes depend on the different management techniques and postoperative functional rehabilitation.

Specifically, the risks and benefits of operative vs. non-operative treatment are still contentious, and the most cost-effective method has not been determined [2].

If the AT is left untreated (or overlooked) for at least 4 weeks, it is classified as chronic or "neglected" Achilles tendon rupture (CATR) [3].

CATR can significantly affect gait due to altered gastrocnemius-soleus complex (GSC) mechanics and muscle atrophy over time [4]. Many surgical techniques have been proposed to address CATR. The flexor hallucis longus (FHL) transfer is a commonly used tendon transfer technique as it works in phase with the Achilles tendon but reduces the first ray's plantar flexion strength [5].

1.1 Anatomy

The AT arises from two muscles: the more superficial gastrocnemius with its medial and lateral heads and the deeper soleus. It is about 15 cm long, 6 mm in diameter at its narrowest point, and changes from a broad fan shape at the top to a cord-like shape at the bottom [2, 6]. At the musculotendinous junction during tendon development, the gastrocnemius-soleus complex rotates internally with the right one rotating counter-clockwise 120° towards its insertion (left clockwise).

The lateral part of the tendon comes from the gastrocnemius muscle, while the soleus muscle makes up the medial part [7].

The insertion site is a special area consisting of a tendon attachment, a layer of hyaline cartilage, and a bone area not covered by periosteum. The AT comprises robust parallel collagen fibres in bundles along the longitudinal axis of the tendon. It is wrapped in a paratenon layer, which creates a lubricated environment for smooth tendon movement [2].

The vascular supply to the AT comes from 3 sources: the surrounding connective tissue, the musculotendinous junction, and the bone-tendon junction. The latter comes from the long and short vincula via the paratenon, mainly from the ventral mesotendon [2, 6].

The posterior zone was considered the watershed zone for the vascularity of the AT and has the poorest blood supply compared to the medial and lateral zones. This hypovascular area has a consistent longitudinal hypovascular shadow directly over the AT [8]. However, this hypovascular theory is no longer supported by current live tissue evidence, as further studies have shown a uniform blood flow in the Achilles tendon including the watershed area [9, 10].

The AT gets its sensory innervation from the muscles it attaches to and the overlying skin nerves, with the sural nerve being the most important [2].

Histologically, tenocytes (mature fibroblasts) and tenoblasts make up 90–95% of the cellular components in the AT. Collagen makes up about 70% of a tendon's dry weight, with 95% being type 1 collagen and a small amount of elastin. The epitenon and paratenon layers are separated by a thin layer of fluid that reduces friction and allows for tendon movement. In a ruptured AT, tenocytes produce more type III collagen than healthy tendons [2, 11]. Type III collagen is less resistant to tensile stress and more prone to rupture [12].

1.2 Biomechanics

With actin and myosin in tenocytes, the AT is optimised to transmit forces from muscles to bones. It is stiff and resilient with high tensile strength and can stretch up to 4% of its original length to handle most physiological loads [2].

The AT can experience uneven stresses due to asynchronous contractions, which can occur due to differences in muscle contributions of the triceps surae components or uncoordinated agonist–antagonist muscle contractions. This uneven stress can lead to differential stress distribution and injury [13].

At rest, the AT has a wavy pattern due to the crimping of collagen fibrils. This pattern disappears when stretched beyond 2%, and the tendon responds linearly to increasing loads. But when the strain exceeds 4% of its normal length, the tendon starts to get damaged, and tensile failure occurs at levels above 8% [2, 14].

2. A cute Achilles tendon rupture

2.1 Aetiology of rupture

2.1.1 Degenerative theory

The degenerative theory outlines three stages of tendon injury as traditionally described: paratenonitis, paratenonitis with tendinosis, and tendinosis itself. Paratenonitis refers to inflammation confined to the paratenon, which thickens and adheres to the tendon. Paratenonitis with tendinosis adds degenerative changes within the tendon structure [6, 15]. Pathological examination of partially and fully ruptured tendons always shows changes associated with tendinosis. These changes are age-related; the ageing process results in morphological changes, fewer organelles in the tenocytes, fewer mucopolysaccharides and glycoproteins, and less diameter and density of collagen fibres [6, 16].

The term tendinopathy has become widely accepted as a comprehensive term that covers the range of tendon disorders, taking the place of older terms like tendinitis and tendinosis, which imply specific inflammatory or degenerative conditions.

Recent perspectives describe tendinopathy as a continuum involving progressive changes in collagen organisation, vascularity, and tenocyte function. Changing collagen cross-linking is one of the new theories explaining tendon deterioration. Advanced glycation end-products (AGEs), which create aberrant covalent bonds between collagen fibres, can build up in ageing and metabolic disorders like diabetes. These cross-links weaken tendon elasticity, lower collagen turnover, and raise tissue stiffness, hence increasing tendon susceptibility to rupture [17, 18].

2.2 Mechanical theory

The mechanical theory relates that the peak incidence occurs in the middle-aged rather than the elderly [2].

A malfunction in the mechanism that protects against excessive or uncoordinated muscle contractions can rupture the site of maximum stress and torsion. Athletes inactive for a while may be most susceptible to this mechanism [2, 19].

Complete rupture can occur in healthy tendons if loaded obliquely at a short initial length with maximum muscle contraction typical of rapid push-offs used in many sports. Therefore, a violent muscle force can cause rupture from incomplete synergism of agonist muscle contractions or inefficient plantaris action [2, 20].

It was shown that AT injury could be due to structural or dynamic disturbances, such as overtraining, functional overpronation, and gastrocnemius-soleus insufficiency. Repeated microtrauma from eccentric loading of fatigued muscle can lead to multiple micro-ruptures and eventual failure beyond a critical point [2, 21].

2.3 Risk factors

Achilles tendon rupture has two various types of risk factors: intrinsic and extrinsic. Intrinsic factors include age, male sex, poor vascularity, stiffness, and conditions such as diabetes mellitus and rheumatoid arthritis. These factors affect tendon healing, quality, and structure. Significant fluctuations in training intensity, poor shoe quality, uneven surfaces, and medications such as corticosteroids and fluoroquinolones are examples of extrinsic variables. The combination of these factors increases the risk, particularly for middle-aged recreational athletes who perform heavy-load exercises and have limited tendon flexibility [2, 6, 14].

2.3.1 Corticosteroids

The risk of AT rupture increases with both systemic and topical corticosteroids administration, especially when combined with other medications, such as fluoroquinolones. Older adults and individuals with preexisting medical conditions are at a higher risk. Corticosteroids alter the structure and function of tendons. They have a direct deleterious effect on human tenocytes, inhibiting their cellular functions and collagen synthesis, which can disrupt tendon structures [2, 22, 23].

2.3.2 Diabetes

Diabetes is a risk factor for AT rupture due to its effects on tendon structure and function. Chronic high blood sugar causes advanced glycation end-products (AGEs) to accumulate, which changes the biomechanical properties of collagen and reduces tendon elasticity and strength [24]. Histology shows increased collagen cross-linking and disorganisation in the tendons of diabetics, making them more prone to degeneration and rupture. Diabetes also causes microvascular changes that impair tendon healing and metabolism, making it more likely to get injured [25, 26].

2.3.3 Fluoroquinolone

Fluoroquinolone antibiotics, such as ciprofloxacin, are associated with the development of Achilles tendinopathy. These treatments can lead to a range of tendon disorders, including ruptures [2, 27].

Fluoroquinolones inhibit the bacterial enzymes topoisomerases II and IV, disrupting DNA synthesis. The inhibition of similar enzymes involved in connective tissue metabolism results in increased expression of matrix metalloproteinases and collagen degradation, reduced cell proliferation, and impaired synthesis of collagen and proteoglycans [28, 29].

2.4 Diagnosis

The assessment of AT ruptures necessitates meticulous history taking, physical examination, and imaging studies to confirm the diagnosis. Typically, the affected individual is a middle-aged male engaged in sports that involve abrupt starting and stopping, such as soccer, tennis, basketball, or badminton [2, 30].

Patients with acute tendon rupture frequently report hearing a popping sound in the posterior leg during ankle dorsiflexion or experiencing a sensation akin to being kicked in the back of the ankle [2, 30].

Three primary mechanisms have been identified for indirect injuries to the AT. Many of these injuries occur when an individual pushes off the weight-bearing forefoot while extending the knee. Others result from sudden, unexpected dorsiflexion of the ankle, such as when an individual slips into a hole, and some are caused by violent dorsiflexion of a plantar-flexed foot, often observed in falls from a height [2, 31].

Signs of a ruptured tendon include plantar flexion weakness and difficulty with weight-bearing ambulation. The clinical examination may reveal oedema and bruising with a palpable gap along the course of the tendon. Physical examinations involve conducting the Thompson test and assessing the ankle's range of motion. The tendon gap can be easily palpated once leg swelling subsides, typically 5–7 days post-injury [1, 6]. The Simmonds–Thompson test is a highly sensitive diagnostic tool for Achilles tendon rupture. It involves the physician squeezing the calf muscle with the patient kneeling in the prone position and observing the movement of the ankle. A lack of ankle plantar flexion is a positive Simmonds–Thompson test result, indicating an AT rupture [32, 33]. However, a negative test result does not necessarily indicate healthy tendons. Another helpful test is the knee flexion test. The patient is again placed in the prone position on the examination couch and flexes both knees to 90°.Greater dorsiflexion of the affected ankle indicates rupture [1, 6].

In some cases, an accurate diagnosis of complete rupture is challenging based solely on physical examination findings. A large hematoma can obscure tendon defects. The plantar flexion power of the extrinsic foot flexors is retained. Moreover, the Simmonds–Thompson test can give false-positive results if the accessory ankle flexors (posterior tibialis, flexor digitorum longus, and flexor hallucis longus muscles) are compressed together with the contents of the superficial posterior leg compartment [6, 34]. Delayed or missed diagnosis of AT ruptures in primary care is relatively common. Inglis et al. reported that 22% of AT ruptures were initially misdiagnosed, highlighting the diagnostic challenges [35].

According to the American Academy of Orthopaedic Surgeons clinical practice guidelines, the diagnosis of an acute AT rupture can be established by two or more of the following physical examination tests: (1) a positive Thompson test, (2) decreased plantar flexion strength, (3) presence of a palpable defect, and (4) increased passive ankle dorsiflexion with gentle manipulation [36].

2.5 Radiological findings

2.5.1 Plain radiography

Most practitioners consider radiography of secondary importance to physical examination. On the lateral radiograph, Kager et al. recognised a triangle filled with fat bordered by the anterior edge of the AT, the back of the tibia, and the upper part of the calcaneus. After a rupture, the anterior edge of the AT moves close to the back of the tibia, resulting in the triangle losing its standard shape [2].

Lateral ankle radiographs are used in treatment planning as they may show a calcific lesions, Haglund prominence, or calcaneus avulsion fractures [34].

Sonography and magnetic resonance imaging are the best imaging techniques for visualising the AT. Each has advantages and disadvantages. Sonography is relatively quick and inexpensive. It is fast, repeatable, and allows for dynamic examination.

However, using the probe and interpreting the images correctly requires much experience. It provides the highest reliability for assessing Achilles tendon thickness and gap size [37, 38].

On the other hand, MRI is more expensive and not typically used for dynamic assessment. However, it is better at detecting incomplete tendon ruptures and chronic degenerative changes. MRI is beneficial in defining the quality of the AT and whether it needs repair. For example, tendon transfer might be a better option for gross degeneration. MRI can also identify the presence of plantaris, which could be used as an adjunct to repair or reconstruction [2, 6].

Imaging modality selection involves multiple considerations, including injury severity, patient medical history, modality availability, and physician preference [1].

In some cases, a combination of imaging modalities might be indicated to confirm the diagnosis and determine the optimal treatment approach [1].

The recommended protocol starts with sonography because it is easy to use, allows for dynamic examination, and is less expensive. If the ultrasound findings are equivocal, an MR study can be performed [6, 39, 40].

2.6 Management

The main goals in treating a ruptured AT are to restore the length and tension of the tendon and maximise its strength and function. There is ongoing debate as to whether operative or non-operative is better [1, 2].

2.7 Non-operative treatment

Non-operative treatment focuses on to ensure proper approximation and alignment of the ruptured tendon ends to facilitate intrinsic healing. Non-operative management should not be misunderstood as an absence of treatment. Validated functional rehabilitation protocols constitute a fundamental component of the conservative management of acute Achilles tendon rupture. These protocols are expected to be effective when applied to informed and cooperative patients [34].

Non-operative treatment varies widely but usually involves immobilisation with either a rigid cast or functional bracing. Initially, the foot is placed in full equinus, and over 8–12 weeks, it is gradually moved to neutral as the ankle allows. The definition of functional (dynamic) rehabilitation varies among researchers and may involve early controlled motion, protected weight-bearing or a combination of both. The methods of protected motion also vary from using a removable rigid boot for a range of motion (ROM) exercises to adjustable, non-removable short-leg orthoses that allow progressive limited ankle movement [41, 42].

The benefits of early motion on tendon healing are well-documented and researched in rat models. Controlled mechanical loading stimulates better tendon healing by promoting stronger tissue remodelling, eventually leading to a stronger tendon callus [43].

A randomised controlled trial conducted by Schepull and Aspenberg showed that early controlled tensional loading significantly improved the mechanical strength of healing human Achilles tendons. This supports the role of early mobilisation in enhancing tendon recovery after rupture [44].

The Swansea Morriston Achilles Rupture Treatment (SMART) protocol was introduced in the United Kingdom 2008 to provide a dedicated management approach for patients with Achilles tendon rupture, and the protocol had subsequent changes [45].

The process starts in the emergency department when a patient presents with an AT rupture, confirmed clinically by using Simmonds test. A non-weight-bearing equinus back slab is applied immediately, and the patient is referred to the fracture clinic for further management. A semi-urgent ultrasound examination is done ideally on the same or the next working day. The ultrasound is crucial as it confirms the diagnosis, specifies the exact location and extent of the rupture, and measures the smallest gap between the tendon ends when the foot is in various equinus positions 20° to 30° plantar flexion [45] .

This information is essential to decide whether the patient will be managed conservatively or surgically [45].

Specific criteria based on ultrasound findings are used to recommend surgery. For example, patients under 55 years old with a rupture in the tendon body and a gap greater than 1 cm on passive plantar flexion are usually advised to have surgery; other patients not meeting these criteria or with specific comorbidities are treated conservatively [45]. The reasoning behind this was that if the tendon heals with a gap exceeding 1 cm, its function is likely to be compromised [45, 46].

Once the decision is made, the ultrasound can also determine the immobilisation position; for example, if the tendon ends overlap when the foot is in full plantar flexion, the ankle is adjusted to a dorsiflexed position to align the tendon ends [45].

Patients managed conservatively are placed in a weight-bearing cast in maximum equinus or a boot for roughly 2 weeks. After this period, they progress to a walking orthosis that allows further reduction of the equinus position. Functional orthoses that permit controlled plantar flexion are used to promote early weight-bearing [45].

All patients are sent to the Achilles tendon clinic, where their rehabilitation is supervised by specialised physiotherapists. The program provides strict rehabilitation protocols that outline a progressive exercise plan for the patients. After the prescribed orthosis is removed, patients shift to physiotherapy at local hospitals and are monitored in the clinic until full activity is achieved [45].

3. Operative management

The operative treatment of a ruptured Achilles tendon can be divided into four types: open repair, percutaneous repair, mini-open repair, and augmentative repair. Surgery is generally recommended for younger patients and those with higher functional demands, such as athletes or individuals with physically demanding occupations, as it may better restore tendon strength and reduce the risk of re-rupture [47].

3.1 Open repair

Open repair is a straightforward end-to-end repair with a long incision to the rupture site, and various suturing techniques can be used to align the tendon ends which can be done by posterior or posteromedial approach [41].

Regardless of the surgical method, getting the tendon back to its original length is crucial to prevent over-lengthening [41].

The posteromedial approach is most commonly used as the medial side of the Achilles tendon is hypervascular. Yepes et al. performed a vascular mapping study of the skin overlying the AT and found the medial zone to have the richest blood supply [48]. They recommended the posteromedial approach for surgical access [48]. This approach is reliable with the patient in the supine position and the surgical limb externally rotated with a beanbag, avoiding the risks and difficulties of a prone position [49]. However, clinically, the choice of the approach does not affect significantly the wound complication rates. A systematic review by Highlander and Greenhagen showed wound complication rates of 7 and 8.3% for midline and posteromedial incisions, respectively [50].

During open repair, a 6–10 cm skin incision is made medial to the Achilles tendon, avoiding the sural nerve.

The debate about the best suture for the AT continues, with the Kessler, Bunnell, and Krakow being the most commonly used. The Kessler is a simple locking loop with moderate tensile strength. The Bunnell suture has longitudinal and transverse elements and even tension distribution. The Krackow is a multi-loop locking suture applied longitudinally with a more even tension distribution. Biomechanical research indicates that suture methods, including the Krackow and Bunnell techniques, can withstand higher loads before failure compared to the Kessler technique. The durability of any repair depends on multiple factors, including the type and thickness of the suture material, the number of strands across the repair site, the complexity of the weaving technique, and the knot configuration and its security. The Krackow or Bunnell techniques offer biomechanical advantages under particular conditions; however, the ultimate repair strength depends on multiple factors that need be adapted to the clinical situation [51, 52].

If the defect is over 3 cm, augmentation, tissue matrix tendon graft transplants, and turndown gastrocnemius muscle flaps might be necessary [47]. Another option is plantaris tendon augmentation; the small diameter of the plantaris tendon limits this technique [53].

However, two prospective randomised trials did not show any augmentation benefit over simple end-to-end repair [54, 55].

The repair length is determined during surgery by comparing it with the intact plantaris tendon; if the plantaris tendon is absent, the dorsiflexion range on the opposite side should be measured before draping or during surgery as a reference [31].

Kou recommend to close of the paratenon over the Achilles tendon as it provides an extra layer of protection in case of wound dehiscence and to avoid adhesions [56].

3.2 Percutaneous repair

Percutaneous repair of AT injuries has been driven by the desire to reduce wound complications, mainly by minimising the incision size and devitalising the surrounding soft tissue. This involves multiple puncture wounds through which a suture is woven across the proximal and distal ends of the tendon. The suture is tied, and the tendon ends are aligned during ankle plantar flexion, However, differences in repair strength and tendon apposition exist, which may affect clinical outcomes [41, 52].

A significant limitation of percutaneous repair is the risk of the sural nerve injury, which can cause sensory disturbances, severe pain, or functional impairment. Earlier studies reported sural nerve injury with percutaneous repair; however, recent studies show a reduction or absence of this complication. This is related to the advances in surgical techniques, particularly the careful identification and protection of the sural nerve through proximal lateral stab incisions [57].

However, Webb and Bannister [58] introduced a percutaneous technique using only three midline skin incisions away from the lateral side of the tendon to protect the sural nerve.

Furthermore, Wagnon and Akayi [59] did a retrospective review of 57 consecutive patients with this modified percutaneous technique and found no neurological damage. Percutaneous repair is considered a good option for elite athletes to allow for prompt return to sporting activities.

Yang et al. [60] undertook a meta-analysis of 12 studies with 815 patients that compared open and percutaneous repairs for acute AT ruptures. They concluded that percutaneous repair had better outcomes in some aspects, including lower rates of deep infections, less time in the operating room, and improved AOFAS scores. However, percutaneous repair was associated with a higher risk of sural nerve injury. No significant difference was observed in re-rupture rates and most functional outcomes. The authors concluded that percutaneous repair may be preferable despite the nerve injury risk [60].

Intraoperative ultrasonography can aid in achieving tendon end apposition and identifying the sural nerve trajectory, thereby reducing the risk of iatrogenic injury during percutaneous repair of the Achilles tendon [61].

3.3 Mini-open repair

The mini-open repair technique provides advantages for AT injuries compared to percutaneous methods. The surgeon can directly visualise tendon apposition while evaluating repair quality and confirming adequate tendon length restoration. This technique increases the contact of the edges of the ruptured tendon [41].

A limited open procedure was developed to combine the advantages of open surgery methods with percutaneous techniques. The surgeon creates a small incision through the skin directly above the rupture point and then bluntly separates the underlying soft tissue. The incision allows for the removal of blood clots and interposed tissue [62].

The mini-open method minimises sural nerve injury better than the percutaneous approach and reduces wound complications more effectively than the classic open technique while delivering adequate initial repair strength [34].

Cho et al. conducted a meta-analysis comparing open repair to percutaneous and mini-open for AT ruptures. The analysis of 26 studies with 1898 patients showed that percutaneous repair had lower infection rates and shorter operative times than open repair, but higher sural nerve injury. Mini-open repair was better across all measures, with better functional scores, lower re-rupture and nerve injury than percutaneous repair, and a lower infection rate than open repair. That mini-open repair provides the optimal combination of safety and effectiveness [63].

A possible drawback of the mini-open technique is that it requires opening the rupture site. This might lead to the removal of the haematoma and the loss of all tendon growth factors and inflammatory mediators. They are theoretically vital for tendon repair, as they promote a complete and more physiological restoration of the ruptured tendon [64].

3.4 Postoperative rehabilitation

Extended immobilisation after surgery is not advisable. Specifically, keeping a limb immobilised in a splint or cast for over 3 weeks should be avoided. The use of a long-leg cast is no longer suggested. Patients should begin full weight-bearing in an orthosis right after surgery or at the latest within 3weeks, and this should continue for 6 to 8 weeks post-surgery. While a removable brace can be used for early range-of-motion exercises, patients should be warned against excessive ankle dorsiflexion [34].

The AAOS guidelines recommend a postoperative plan supporting early, protected weight-bearing in a protective device facilitating movement. The cast is taken off during the first postoperative visit, and the wound is checked. If the incision has healed, sutures are removed, and the patient is fitted with a brace that includes removable heel wedges. The patient can gradually increase weight-bearing as tolerated while wearing the brace. After 3 weeks, the heel wedges in the brace are slowly removed for 2 to 3 weeks. After 1 week of walking in the brace without wedges, the patient begins walking without the brace [56].

Massen et al. conducted a meta-analysis of 20 randomised controlled trials comparing different postoperative rehabilitation protocols following surgical repair of acute AT rupture. They found that early functional rehabilitation, including early weight-bearing and ankle mobilisation, was associated with lower re-rupture and complications and quicker return to work and sport [65].

3.5 Biological adjuncts

The pursuit of better outcomes in acute AT repairs has led to the exploration of biological augmentation.

Fibrin sealant, a product made from blood, allows for anatomical reconstruction with less soft tissue damage than suture repair [47].

Knobe et al. compared percutaneous suturing and open fibrin glue application for acute AT ruptures. They found that both methods had similar functional outcomes and complication rates, and they concluded that open fibrin glueing is a viable alternative to percutaneous repair for acute AT ruptures [66].

Platelet-rich fibrin matrix (PRF), a second-generation platelet concentrate obtained from blood centrifugation, contains a complex array of signalling factors that promote tendon cell proliferation and healing. These factors stimulate type I collagen production and healthy tissue growth. PRF has been investigated as a treatment for AT rupture, healing, and functional recovery [46, 67].

Alviti et al. studied the biomechanical outcomes of AT repair with and without PRF matrix augmentation in a retrospective study with gait analysis 6 months post-op. Patients who received PRF augmentation had ankle biomechanics closer to healthy controls. These findings support the PRF role as an adjunct in tendon repair [68].

Sánchez et al. studied autologous platelet-rich fibrin (PRGF) in Achilles tendon repair. They found it accelerated recovery, allowing for earlier return to motion and training compared to standard repair. The PRGF group had fewer complications and more physiological tendon healing, as seen in the ultrasound assessment. They concluded that PRGF is a promising adjunct to improve healing and functional outcomes after surgical repair [67].

Mesenchymal stem cells (MSCS) contribute to tendon healing through their anti-apoptotic effects, differentiation into tenocytes, and production of signalling factors. MSCS also increase collagen types I and III production, which is important for tendon strength and flexibility [46, 69].

They downregulate matrix metalloproteinase-9 (MMP-9), which is involved in tissue degradation. This reduces inflammation and creates a favourable environment for tendon healing. Additionally, MSCS promote neovascularisation and cell proliferation, which are crucial for tissue repair [69].

Stein et al. [70] reported good results in patients with AT ruptures who underwent open AT repair with bone marrow aspirate concentrate (BMAC), which is mainly composed of MSCS and growth factors. There were no ruptures in the cohort of 27 patients, and most returned to sports in 6 months with a low complication rate. These findings concluded that BMAC may be a safe and effective adjunct. However, further research is needed [70].

However, more study is required as present meta-analyses, and systematic reviews have not yet found substantial, evidence-based support for every kind of biological adjuncts [65, 67, 70].

3.6 Chronic achilles ruptures

There is no agreed-upon definition for late, chronic or neglected rupture, but different authors have used these terms in different study groups. However, a rupture is generally considered neglected or chronic if left untreated for more than 4 weeks post-injury [3, 71].

The body responds to an acute AT with an organised connective tissue response. Nevertheless, if the tendon ends are not at the correct resting length, a regular fascicular arrangement may not develop [69]. Non-fascicular scar tissue is stretchy and can elongate, reducing the efficiency of the gastrocnemius-soleus complex (GSC) and resulting in push-off weakness. The retracted proximal Achilles tendon stump often adheres to the ventral flexor hallucis longus (FHL) tendon, and the distal portion can be extensively frayed [4, 72].

3.7 Diagnosis

Chronic AT ruptures usually present as a result of a misdiagnosed, neglected, or unrecognised acute rupture [72].

When a patient has a chronic rupture, the pain and swelling often subside, and the gap between the tendon ends is filled with fibrous tissue. This fibrous tissue is predominantly non-fascicular scar tissue, characterised by a lack of the organised collagen architecture found in a healthy tendon. It is mechanically inferior, being more elastic and susceptible to elongation, which results in decreased tension within the gastrocnemius-soleus complex and a consequent reduction in push-off strength during gait [4, 72].

In addition, active plantar flexion, although weak, may be possible through the actions of the tibialis posterior, flexor hallucis longus, flexor digitorum longus, and peroneal muscles. These residual functions may make it difficult to confirm a correct diagnosis through clinical examination alone [4, 72].

A high index of suspicion is required, and a range of special tests and investigations can aid in accurate diagnosis [4].

3.8 Clinical examination

On inspection, a visible gap may be observed at the rupture site. The calf muscles may have been wasted. The long toe flexors may accommodate the lack of function of the gastrocnemius—soleus complex, producing clawing of the toes and an apparently higher medial arch of the foot [72].

A comprehensive neurovascular examination should be conducted, accompanied by an evaluation of the skin for any contracture at the site of the chronic rupture [4].

Clinical tests for assessing the integrity of the Achilles tendon include the Simmonds–Thompson test [23, 33].

The Matles test can also be performed with the patient in the prone position. The knees are flexed to 90°. The ankle on the ruptured side will assume a more dorsiflexed position than the normal side [73]. This is due to the absence of normal tension under which the tendon connects the gastrocnemius-soleus complex to the calcaneus; hence, the effects of gravity make the foot dorsiflex more on the injured side [73].

The O'Brien needle test [74] is also performed with the patient in the prone position. A hypodermic needle is inserted off the midline 10 cm proximal to the calcaneal insertion of the AT, such that its tip lies within the tendon substance. The examiner manually moves the ankle through plantarflexion and dorsiflexion while observing the movement of the needle hup. If the needle hup moves, it indicates the tendon segment between the needle and calcaneus is intact; otherwise, a rupture is suspected. If, on dorsiflexion, the pin moves so that it points proximally, the tendon area between the pin and calcaneus is presumed to be intact; otherwise, a rupture is probable [74].

3.9 Imaging

Lateral X-rays can help to identify a suspected chronic rupture of the AT. Loss of the normal contour of the Achilles tendon and definition of the Kager triangle can be seen. Changes in the AT indicate that previous tendinopathy may have contributed to the overall deterioration of the tendon and its attachment, and this can be seen from a prominent Haglund's prominence or significant calcification along the AT or at its calcaneal insertion [4, 72].

Ultrasonography has been shown to be effective in diagnosing stages of neo-vascularisation and abnormal tendon structure in chronic Achilles tendinopathy. Echogenicity can vary depending on the chronicity of the rupture. With a high frequency probe, ultrasonography can further detail an Achilles tear, showing the morphology of the tendon ends and loss of the normal hypoechogenicity of the tendon [72, 75].

MRI, especially sagittal sequences, can give a full picture of the AT including the chronic rupture pattern. In chronic rupture, sagittal T2 weighted sequences will show a mixed signal with tendon thickening, T1 sequences will be dark, and all sequences will show discontinuity, sometimes with scar tissue between the tendon ends [4, 72].

3.10 Management

The management of chronic Achilles tendon ruptures presents significant challenges. The tendon ends are often retracted and exhibit atrophic characteristics.

3.11 Non-operative management

Surgery is usually recommended for chronic Achilles tendon ruptures, but non-operative management may be an option for some patients. This is especially for elderly patients with low demand or unfit for surgery due to poor soft tissue condition, poor vascular supply, active infection, heavy smoker, or comorbidities that increase surgical risk. An ankle foot orthosis can help improve gait stability and overall function in these cases [4, 72].

3.12 Operative treatment of chronic Achilles tendon ruptures

Surgery is helpful in most cases as it aims to restore the anatomical length and tension of the gastrocnemius-soleus complex (GSC) and, therefore, push-off strength and functional mobility [4, 72].

3.12.1 Preoperative considerations

The choice of surgical technique is determined by several factors, including the size of the tendon defect post-debridement, the quality and blood supply of the remaining tendon tissue, the location of the rupture and patient-specific factors such as comorbidities, activity level, and the integrity of the soft tissue envelope. Preoperative MRI and intraoperative evaluation are essential for surgical planning, especially for measuring the gap after removing nonviable tissue [4, 72, 76].

The Myerson protocol categorises chronic AT injuries based on defect size. Lesions with gaps less than 2 cm are directly repaired. Gaps 2–5 cm are repaired with V-Y advancement and sometimes tendon transfer if needed. Gaps greater than 5 cm are primarily repaired with tendon transfer and V-Y lengthening if needed [72, 77].

3.12.2 Primary repair for small defects

Primary end-to-end repair is possible and suitable for tendon gaps less than 2–3 cm, typically Myerson type I ruptures. Mobilising the tendon stumps and applying gentle longitudinal traction often suffice to make the stumps to be approximated. Additional procedures, such as posterior compartment fasciotomy, may improve vascularity and close the paratenon [4, 72]. Studies have shown a good return to pre-injury activity level in appropriately selected patients in this category [78].

3.12.3 Reconstruction for moderate defects (2–5 cm)

Moderate defects as in cases of Myerson type II require more complex surgical solutions due to tendon loss and muscle-tendon unit (MTU) contracture. V-Y gastrocnemius fascial advancement is a common reconstructive technique. This involves making an inverted V incision in the proximal aponeurosis, which is then advanced and sutured in a Y configuration to lengthen the tendon. Although it is an effective procedure, care must be taken not to overlengthen the tendon, which can compromise plantar flexion strength [4, 72].

The Achilles tendon turn-down flap is another well-established method for this purpose. In this approach, a centrally based strip of the proximal tendon is reflected distally to bridge the gap. This technique is often augmented with a tendon transfer. Mulier et al. found better results when combining the turn-down flap and FHL tendon transfer [79].

3.12.4 Tendon transfers

Tendon transfers are significant in managing chronic ruptures if the Achilles tendon is not amenable to repair. The FHL transfer is the most studied and preferred option. This tendon and its pull strength are appropriately positioned compared to the AT. The musculotendinous unit has a good blood supply in the belly of the muscle [4, 72]. Harvesting can be short or long, the long harvest, which includes obtaining the tendon at the knot of Henry or its distal insertion, offers length for double-limb reconstructions [80].

The Peroneus brevis (PB) transfer is a less invasive option for defects less than 5 cm. Although there are concerns about decreased eversion strength, clinical studies have shown good functional outcomes with minimal effect on gait and daily activities [81].

3.12.5 Reconstruction for large defects (>5 cm)

Large defects are beyond the bridging capacity of local repair techniques. In these cases, free tendon autografts such as gracilis, semitendinosus, or quadriceps tendons are used. These grafts are looped and woven through the proximal and distal stumps or secured via calcaneal bone tunnels [4, 72].

Allograft reconstruction, especially with the AT, with a calcaneal bone block, is another option when autograft harvesting is not possible or inadequate. These grafts provide structural support and avoid donor site complications. However, concerns about cost, disease transmission, immune response, and integration remain [82].

3.12.6 Synthetic augmentation

Synthetic scaffolds and materials such as Dacron, polyester tapes, dermal matrices, and degradable polymers have been suggested as alternatives and supplements. While biomechanical studies have shown good initial tensile strength, clinical data are limited, and issues with infection and soft tissue irritation persist. Therefore, synthetic materials are generally reserved for complex salvage cases [4, 72, 83].

3.12.7 Postoperative management and outcomes

Rehabilitation protocols are customised based on the complexity of the repair. Early functional bracing with limited dorsiflexion, protected weight-bearing, and gradual loading is common. Full functional recovery may take 9–12 months. Although returning to high-level activity is possible, many patients will have ongoing calf strength and volume deficits, especially after extensive reconstruction or tendon transfer [4, 72].

4. Conclusion

AT tears can seriously impact a patient's mobility and lifestyle. This chapter has discussed the anatomy of tendons, mechanisms of injury, diagnosis, and treatment. Both non-operative and operative options can be effective, especially when accompanied by prompt and structured rehabilitation. Minimal invasive surgery and biological treatment techniques are promising in improving results while minimising complications.

The management of chronic ruptures tends to be more complicated and may require tendon transfer or more reconstructive surgeries. These challenging cases highlight the value of early, accurate diagnosis, and timely treatment strategy initiation.

Comprehensive comparative studies focusing on treatment modalities and their long-term impacts are necessary to improve the care provided to patients with Achilles tendon injuries.

Author details

Sedeek M. Mosaid*, Ashok Marudanayagam, Rizwan Shahid and Mohamed Elnemr
Department of Trauma and Orthopaedics, United Lincolnshire Hospitals NHS Trust, Lincoln, United Kingdom

*Address all correspondence to: sedeeko2000@hotmail.com

References

[1] Wang CC, Chen PY, Yang KC, Wang CL, Chen IH. Current treatment concepts for Achilles tendon rupture [internet]. Tzu Chi Medical Journal. 2024;**36**(1):46. Available from: https://journals.lww.com/tcmj/fulltext/2024/36010/current_treatment_concepts_for_achilles_tendon.5.aspx?context=latestarticles

[2] Thevendran G, Sarraf KM, Patel NK, Sadri A, Rosenfeld P. The ruptured Achilles tendon: A current overview from biology of rupture to treatment [internet]. Musculoskeletal Surgery. 2013;**97**(1):9-20. Available from: https://link.springer.com/article/10.1007/s12306-013-0251-6

[3] Flint JH, Wade AM, Giuliani J, Rue JP. Defining the terms acute and chronic in orthopaedic sports injuries. The American Journal of Sports Medicine. 2013;**42**(1):235-241. DOI: 10.1177/0363546513490656

[4] Schweitzer KM, Dekker TJ, Adams SB. Chronic Achilles ruptures: Reconstructive options. The Journal of the American Academy of Orthopaedic Surgeons. 2018;**26**(21):753-763. DOI: 10.5435/JAAOS-D-17-00158

[5] Fischer S, Kutscher R, Gramlich Y, Klug A, Hoffmann R, Manegold S. Secondary reconstruction of chronic Achilles tendon rupture: Flexor hallucis longus transfer versus plantaris longus augmentation. International Orthopaedics. 2021;**45**(9):2323-2330. DOI: 10.1007/s00264-021-05128-9

[6] Saltzman CL, Tearse DS. Achilles tendon injuries. Journal of the American Academy of Orthopaedic Surgeons. 1998;**6**(5):316-325. DOI: 10.5435/00124635-199809000-00007

[7] Rufai A, Ralphs JR, Benjamin M. Structure and histopathology of the insertional region of the human Achilles tendon. Journal of Orthopaedic Research. 1995;**13**(4):585-593. DOI: 10.1002/jor.1100130414

[8] Saxena A, Bareither D. Magnetic resonance and cadaveric findings of the "watershed band" of Achilles tendon. The Journal of Foot and Ankle Surgery. 2001;**40**(3):132-136. DOI: 10.1016/s1067-2516(01)80078-8

[9] Boushel R, Langberg H, Green S, Skovgaard D, Bülow J, Kjaer M. Blood flow and oxygenation in peritendinous tissue and calf muscle during dynamic exercise in humans. The Journal of Physiology. 2000;**524**(1):305-313. DOI: 10.1111/j.1469-7793.2000.t01-2-00305.x

[10] Kubo K, Ikebukuro T, Tsunoda N, Kanehisa H. Noninvasive measures of blood volume and oxygen saturation of human Achilles tendon by red laser lights. Acta Physiologica. 2008;**193**(3):257-264. DOI: 10.1111/j.1748-1716.2008.01841.x

[11] Maffulli N, Ewen SWB, Waterston SW, Reaper J, Barrass V. Tenocytes from ruptured and tendinopathic Achilles tendons produce greater quantities of type III collagen than tenocytes from normal Achilles tendons: An in vitro model of human tendon healing. The American Journal of Sports Medicine. 2000;**28**(4):499-505. DOI: 10.1177/03635465000280040901

[12] Liu SH, Yang RS, al-Shaikh R, Lane JM. Collagen in tendon, ligament, and bone healing. A current review. Clinical Orthopaedics and Related Research. 1995;**318**:265-278

[13] Arndt AN, Komi PV, Brüggemann GP, Lukkariniemi J. Individual muscle contributions to the in vivo Achilles tendon force. Clinical Biomechanics (Bristol). 1998;**13**(7):532-541. DOI: 10.1016/s0268-0033(98)00032-1

[14] Mafulli N. Current concepts review - rupture of the Achilles tendon. The Journal of Bone & Joint Surgery. 1999;**81**(7):1019-1036

[15] Järvinen M, Józsa L, Kannus P, Järvinen TL, Kvist M, Leadbetter W. Histopathological findings in chronic tendon disorders. Scandinavian Journal of Medicine & Science in Sports. 1997;**7**(2):86-95. DOI: 10.1111/j.1600-0838.1997.tb00124.x

[16] Kannus P, Józsa L. Histopathological changes preceding spontaneous rupture of a tendon. A controlled study of 891 patients. The Journal of Bone & Joint Surgery. 1991;**73**(10):1507-1525

[17] Steinmann S, Pfeifer CG, Brochhausen C, Docheva D. Spectrum of tendon pathologies: Triggers, trails and end-state. International Journal of Molecular Sciences [Internet]. 2020;**21**(3):844. DOI: 10.3390/ijms21030844

[18] Paoloni J. Current Strategy in the Treatment of Achilles Tendinopathy. In: Tendon Surgery – Innovations and Challenges. Rijeka, Croatia: InTechOpen; 2012. Available from: https://www.intechopen.com/books/achilles-tendon/achilles-tendon-injury-management

[19] Inglis AE, Sculco TP. Surgical repair of ruptures of the tendo Achillis. Clinical Orthopaedics and Related Research. 1981;**156**:160-169

[20] Barfred T. Experimental rupture of the Achilles tendon: Comparison of various types of experimental rupture in rats. Acta Orthopaedica Scandinavica. 1971;**42**(6):528-543. DOI: 10.3109/17453677108989070

[21] Clement DB, Taunton JE, Smart GW. Achilles tendinitis and peritendinitis: Etiology and treatment. The American Journal of Sports Medicine. 1984;**12**(3):179-184. DOI: 10.1177/036354658401200301

[22] Kennedy JC, Willis RB. The effects of local steroid injections on tendons: A biomechanical and microscopic correlative study. The American Journal of Sports Medicine. 1976;**4**(1):11-21. DOI: 10.1177/036354657600400103

[23] Wong MWN, Tang YN, Fu SC, Lee KM, Chan KM. Triamcinolone suppresses human tenocyte cellular activity and collagen synthesis. Clinical Orthopaedics and Related Research. 2004;**421**:277-281. DOI: 10.1097/01.blo.0000118184.83983.65

[24] Zellers JA, Eekhoff JD, Walk RE, Hastings MK, Tang SY, Lake SP. Human Achilles tendon mechanical behavior is more strongly related to collagen disorganization than advanced glycation end-products content. Scientific Reports. 2021;**11**(1):24147. DOI: 10.1038/s41598-021-03574-4

[25] Nichols AEC, Oh I, Loiselle AE. Effects of type II diabetes mellitus on tendon homeostasis and healing. Journal of Orthopaedic Research. 2020;**38**(1):13-22. DOI: 10.1002/jor.24388

[26] Sankova MV, Beeraka NM, Oganesyan MV, Rizaeva NA, Sankov AV, Shelestova OS, et al. Recent developments in Achilles tendon risk-analyzing rupture factors for enhanced injury prevention and clinical guidance: Current implications of regenerative medicine. Journal of Orthopaedic

Translation. 2024;**49**:289-307. DOI: 10.1016/j.jot.2024.08.024

[27] Royer RJ, Pierfitte C, Netter P. Features of tendon disorders with fluoroquinolones. Thérapie. 1994;**49**(1):75-76

[28] Baik S, Lau J, Huser V, McDonald CJ. Association between tendon ruptures and use of fluoroquinolone, and other oral antibiotics: A 10-year retrospective study of 1 million US senior Medicare beneficiaries. BMJ Open. 2020;**10**(12):e034844. DOI: 10.1136/bmjopen-2019-034844

[29] Nyyssönen T, Lantto I, Lüthje P, Selander T, Kröger H. Drug treatments associated with Achilles tendon rupture. A case-control study involving 1118 Achilles tendon ruptures. Scandinavian Journal of Medicine & Science in Sports. 2018;**28**(12):2625-2629. DOI: 10.1111/sms.13281

[30] Hattrup SJ, Johnson KA. A review of ruptures of the Achilles tendon. Foot & Ankle. 1985;**6**(1):34-38. DOI: 10.1177/107110078500600107

[31] Hess GW. Achilles tendon rupture: A review of etiology, population, anatomy, risk factors, and injury prevention. Foot & Ankle Specialist. 2009;**3**(1):29-32. DOI: 10.1177/1938640009355191

[32] Simmonds FA. The diagnosis of the ruptured Achilles tendon. The Practitioner. 1957;**179**(1069):56-58

[33] Thompson TC. A test for rupture of the tendo Achillis. Acta Orthopaedica Scandinavica. 1962;**32**(1-4):461-465. DOI: 10.3109/17453676208989608

[34] Park SH, Lee HS, Young KW, Seo SG. Treatment of acute Achilles tendon rupture. Clinics in Orthopedic Surgery. 2020;**12**(1):1-8. DOI: 10.4055/cios.2020.12.1.1

[35] Inglis AE, Scott WN, Sculco TP, Patterson AH. Ruptures of the tendo Achillis. An objective assessment of surgical and non-surgical treatment. The Journal of Bone & Joint Surgery. 1976;**58**(7):990-993

[36] Chiodo CP, Glazebrook M, Bluman EM, Cohen BE, Femino JE, Giza E, et al. Diagnosis and treatment of acute Achilles tendon rupture. The Journal of the American Academy of Orthopaedic Surgeons. 2010;**18**(8):503-510. DOI: 10.5435/00124635-201008000-00007

[37] Bleakney RR, Tallon C, Wong JK, Lim KP, Maffulli N. Long-term ultrasonographic features of the Achilles tendon after rupture. Clinical Journal of Sport Medicine. 2002;**12**(5):273-278. DOI: 10.1097/00042752-200209000-00003

[38] Kälebo P, Allenmark C, Peterson L, Swärd L. Diagnostic value of ultrasonography in partial ruptures of the Achilles tendon. The American Journal of Sports Medicine. 1992;**20**(4):378-381. DOI: 10.1177/036354659202000402

[39] Dams OC, Reininga IHF, Gielen JL, van den Akker-Scheek I, Zwerver J. Imaging modalities in the diagnosis and monitoring of Achilles tendon ruptures: A systematic review. Injury. 2017;**48**(11):2383-2399. DOI: 10.1016/j.injury.2017.09.013

[40] Margetić P, Miklić D, Rakić-Ersek V, Doko Z, Lubina ZI, Brkljacić B. Comparison of ultrasonographic and intraoperative findings in Achilles tendon rupture. Collegium Antropologicum. 2007;**31**(1):279-284

[41] Kadakia AR, Dekker RG, Ho BS. Acute Achilles tendon ruptures: An

update on treatment. Journal of the American Academy of Orthopaedic Surgeons. 2017;**25**(1):23-31. DOI: 10.5435/JAAOS-D-15-00187

[42] Neumayer F, Mouhsine E, Arlettaz Y, Gremion G, Wettstein M, Crevoisier X. A new conservative-dynamic treatment for the acute ruptured Achilles tendon. Archives of Orthopaedic and Trauma Surgery. 2010;**130**(3):363-368. DOI: 10.1007/s00402-009-0865-1

[43] Hammerman M, Aspenberg P, Eliasson P. Microtrauma stimulates rat Achilles tendon healing via an early gene expression pattern similar to mechanical loading. Journal of Applied Physiology. 1985;**116**(1):54-60. DOI: 10.1152/japplphysiol.00741.2013

[44] Schepull T, Aspenberg P. Early controlled tension improves the material properties of healing human Achilles tendons after ruptures: A randomized trial. The American Journal of Sports Medicine. 2013;**41**(11):2550-2557. DOI: 10.1177/0363546513501785

[45] Hutchison AM, Topliss C, Beard D, Evans RM, Williams P. The treatment of a rupture of the Achilles tendon using a dedicated management programme. The Bone & Joint Journal. 2015;**97-B**(4):510-515. DOI: 10.1302/0301-620X.97B4.35314

[46] Costa ML, Logan K, Heylings D, Donell ST, Tucker K. The effect of Achilles tendon lengthening on ankle dorsiflexion: A cadaver study. Foot & Ankle International. 2006;**27**(6):414-417. DOI: 10.1177/107110070602700605

[47] Yang X, Meng H, Quan Q, Peng J, Lu S, Wang A. Management of acute Achilles tendon ruptures: A review. Bone & Joint Research. 2018;7(10):561-569. DOI: 10.1302/2046-3758.710.BJR-2018-0004.R2

[48] Yepes H, Tang M, Geddes C, Glazebrook M, Morris SF, Stanish WD. Digital vascular mapping of the integument about the Achilles tendon. The Journal of Bone and Joint Surgery. 2010;**92**(5):1215-1220. DOI: 10.2106/JBJS.I.00743

[49] Tan GJ, Kadakia AR, Jeng CL. Supine patient positioning during repair of Achilles tendon rupture. Foot & Ankle International. 2009;**30**(11):1124-1125. DOI: 10.3113/FAI.2009.1124

[50] Highlander P, Greenhagen RM. Wound complications with posterior midline and posterior medial leg incisions: A systematic review. Foot & Ankle Specialist. 2011;**4**(6):361-369. DOI: 10.1177/1938640011418488

[51] Yammine K, Assi C. Efficacy of repair techniques of the Achilles tendon: A meta-analysis of human cadaveric biomechanical studies. The Foot. 2017;**30**:13-20. DOI: 10.1016/j.foot.2016.09.006

[52] McCoy BW, Haddad SL. The strength of Achilles tendon repair: A comparison of three suture techniques in human cadaver tendons. Foot & Ankle International. 2010;**31**(8):701-705. DOI: 10.3113/FAI.2010.0701

[53] Lynn TA. Repair of the torn Achilles tendon, using the plantaris tendon as a reinforcing membrane. The Journal of Bone and Joint Surgery. 1966;**48**(2):268-272

[54] Heikkinen J, Lantto I, Flinkkilä T, Ohtonen P, Pajala A, Siira P, et al. Augmented compared with nonaugmented surgical repair after total Achilles rupture: Results of a prospective randomized trial with thirteen or more years of follow-up. The Journal of Bone and Joint Surgery. 2016;**98**(2):85-92. DOI: 10.2106/JBJS.O.00496

[55] Pajala A, Kangas J, Siira P, Ohtonen P, Leppilahti J. Augmented compared with nonaugmented surgical repair of a fresh total Achilles tendon rupture. A prospective randomized study. The Journal of Bone and Joint Surgery. 2009;**91**(5):1092-1100. DOI: 10.2106/JBJS.G.01089

[56] Kou J. AAOS clinical practice guideline: Acute Achilles tendon rupture. The Journal of the American Academy of Orthopaedic Surgeons. 2010;**18**(8):511-513. DOI: 10.5435/00124635-201008000-00008

[57] Majewski M, Rohrbach M, Czaja S, Ochsner P. Avoiding sural nerve injuries during percutaneous Achilles tendon repair. The American Journal of Sports Medicine. 2006;**34**(5):793-798. DOI: 10.1177/0363546505283266

[58] Webb JM, Bannister GC. Percutaneous repair of the ruptured tendo Achillis. The Journal of Bone and Joint Surgery. 1999;**81**(5):877-880. DOI: 10.1302/0301-620x.81b5.9784

[59] Wagnon R, Akayi M. The Webb-Bannister percutaneous technique for acute Achilles' tendon ruptures: A functional and MRI assessment. The Journal of Foot and Ankle Surgery. 2005;**44**(6):437-444. DOI: 10.1053/j.jfas.2005.07.015

[60] Yang B, Liu Y, Kan S, Zhang D, Xu H, Liu F, et al. Outcomes and complications of percutaneous versus open repair of acute Achilles tendon rupture: A meta-analysis. International Journal of Surgery. 2017;**40**:178-186. DOI: 10.1016/j.ijsu.2017.03.021

[61] Cross AG, Khalil LS, Tomlinson M, Tramer JS, Makhni EC, Cox BA. Percutaneous Achilles tendon repair using ultrasound guidance: An intraoperative ultrasound technique. Arthroscopy Techniques. 2023;**12**(2):e173-e180. DOI: 10.1016/j.eats.2022.10.006

[62] Keller A, Ortiz C, Wagner E, Wagner P, Mococain P. Mini-open tenorrhaphy of acute Achilles tendon ruptures: Medium-term follow-up of 100 cases. The American Journal of Sports Medicine. 2014;**42**(3):731-736. DOI: 10.1177/0363546513511418

[63] Cho BK, Kim JJ, Choi CH, Kim JB, Choi YS, Kim TH. Comparison of open, percutaneous, and minimally invasive surgical repair for acute Achilles tendon rupture: A meta-analysis of randomized controlled trials. Knee Surgery, Sports Traumatology, Arthroscopy. 2024;**32**(2):650-665. DOI: 10.1007/s00167-023-07412-4

[64] Wagner E, Wagner P, Keller A, Zanolli D, Ortiz C. Minimally invasive Achilles tendon repair. In: Scuedri G, Tria A, editors. Minimally Invasive Surgery in Orthopedics. Cham: Springer; 2016. pp. 1015-1024. DOI: 10.1007/978-3-319-34109-5_99

[65] Massen FK, Shoap S, Vosseller JT, Fan W, Usseglio J, Boecker W, et al. Rehabilitation following operative treatment of acute Achilles tendon ruptures: A systematic review and meta-analysis. EFORT Open Reviews. 2022;**7**(10):680-691. DOI: 10.1530/EOR-22-0072

[66] Knobe M, Gradl G, Klos K, Corsten J, Dienstknecht T, Rath B, et al. Is percutaneous suturing superior to open fibrin gluing in acute Achilles tendon rupture? International Orthopaedics. 2015;**39**(3):535-542. DOI: 10.1007/s00264-014-2615-4

[67] Sánchez M, Anitua E, Azofra J, Andía I, Padilla S, Mujika I. Comparison of surgically repaired Achilles tendon

tears using platelet-rich fibrin matrices. The American Journal of Sports Medicine. 2007;**35**(2):245-251. DOI: 10.1177/0363546506294078

[68] Alviti F, Gurzì M, Santilli V, Paoloni M, Padua R, Bernetti A, et al. Achilles tendon open surgical treatment with platelet-rich fibrin matrix augmentation: Biomechanical evaluation. The Journal of Foot and Ankle Surgery. 2017;**56**(3):581-585. DOI: 10.1053/j.jfas.2017.01.039

[69] Chailakhyan RK, Kon E, Shekhter AB, Ivannikov SV, Telpukhov VI, Grosheva AG, et al. Autologous bone marrow-derived mesenchymal stem cells provide complete regeneration in a rabbit model of the Achilles tendon bundle rupture. International Orthopaedics. 2021;**45**(12):3263-3276. DOI: 10.1007/s00264-021-05168-1

[70] Stein BE, Stroh DA, Schon LC. Outcomes of acute Achilles tendon rupture repair with bone marrow aspirate concentrate augmentation. International Orthopaedics. 2015;**39**(5):901-905. DOI: 10.1007/s00264-015-2725-7

[71] Bendall S. Chronic tendo Achilles injuries: A management rationale. Orthopaedics and Traumatology. 2018;**32**(6):382-387. DOI: 10.1016/j.mporth.2018.09.013

[72] Maffulli N, Ajis A. Management of chronic ruptures of the Achilles tendon. The Journal of Bone & Joint Surgery. 2008;**90**(6):1348-1360. DOI: 10.2106/jbjs.g.01241

[73] Matles AL. Rupture of the tendo Achilles: Another diagnostic sign. Bulletin of the Hospital for Joint Diseases. 1975;**36**(1):48-51

[74] O'Brien T. The needle test for complete rupture of the Achilles tendon. The Journal of Bone & Joint Surgery. 1984;**66**(7):1099-1101

[75] de Vos R-J, Weir A, Cobben LPJ, Tol JL. The value of power Doppler ultrasonography in Achilles tendinopathy: A prospective study. The American Journal of Sports Medicine. 2007;**35**(10):1696-1701. DOI: 10.1177/0363546507303116

[76] Den Hartog BD. Surgical strategies: Delayed diagnosis or neglected Achilles' tendon ruptures. Foot & Ankle International. 2008;**29**(4):456-463. DOI: 10.3113/fai.2008.0456

[77] Myerson MS. Achilles tendon ruptures. Instructional Course Lectures. 1999;**48**:219-230

[78] Porter DA, Mannarino FP, Snead D, Gabel SJ, Ostrowski M. Primary repair without augmentation for early neglected Achilles tendon ruptures in the recreational athlete. Foot & Ankle International. 1997;**18**(9):557-564. DOI: 10.1177/107110079701800905

[79] Mulier T, Pienaar H, Dereymaeker G, Reynders P, Broos P. The management of chronic Achilles tendon ruptures: Gastrocnemius turn down flap with or without flexor hallucis longus transfer. Foot and Ankle Surgery. 2003;**9**(3):151-156. DOI: 10.1016/S1268-7731(03)00048-1

[80] Wapner KL, Pavlock GS, Hecht PJ, Naselli F, Walther R. Repair of chronic Achilles tendon rupture with flexor hallucis longus tendon transfer. Foot & Ankle. 1993;**14**(8):443-449. DOI: 10.1177/107110079301400803

[81] Maffulli N, Spiezia F, Longo UG, Denaro V. Less-invasive reconstruction of chronic Achilles tendon ruptures using a peroneus brevis tendon transfer. The American Journal of Sports

Medicine. 2010;**38**(11):2304-2312. DOI: 10.1177/0363546510376619

[82] Haraguchi N, Bluman EM, Myerson MS. Reconstruction of chronic Achilles tendon disorders with Achilles tendon allograft. Techniques in Foot & Ankle Surgery. 2005;**4**(3):154-159. DOI: 10.1097/01.btf.0000177228.45213.5d

[83] Parsons JR, Weiss AB, Schenk RS, Alexander H, Pavlisko F. Long-term follow-up of Achilles tendon repair with an absorbable polymer carbon fiber composite. Foot & Ankle. 1989;**9**(4):179-184. DOI: 10.1177/107110078900900406

Chapter 7

Wound Healing and Management

Tawheed Ahmad

Abstract

The wound healing process consists of four phases: the hemostasis phase, the inflammatory phase, the fibro-proliferative phase, and the remodeling phase. Wounds may heal either by primary, secondary, or through delayed primary mechanism. Wound healing can be affected by various factors, which include a history of smoking, any drug intake, local wound factors, as well as systemic, genetic, and local wound factors. Excessive scarring can lead to either hypertrophic scars or keloid formation. Currently, there are various modalities for the management of diverse types of wounds, which may, in addition, include the use of wound healing adjuncts like hyperbaric oxygen, stem cells, amnion/chorion allograft, and vacuum-assisted closure (VAC).

Keywords: wound, wound healing process, phases of wound healing, factors affecting wound healing, wound management, hypertrophied scar, keloids, scar management, types of wound dressing, wound healing adjuncts

1. Introduction

Wound healing leads to the restoration of tissue integrity by closely integrated processes [1]. It involves an intricate interplay between cellular components, biochemical mediators, and extracellular matrix (ECM) remodeling. Understanding wound healing is crucial for optimizing patient outcomes, particularly in chronic wounds, burns, surgical wounds, and traumatic injuries. This chapter discusses a comprehensive mechanism of healing, influencing factors, and management of several types of wounds.

2. Phases of wound healing

The wound healing process is divided into four overlapping phases [2]:

1. Hemostasis phase (immediately to a few hours)

2. Inflammatory phase (1st to 6th day)

3. Fibro-proliferative phase (4th day to 3rd week)

4. Maturation/remodeling phase (3rd week to 1 year) [3]

2.1 Hemostasis phase (immediately to a few hours)

This consists of two processes: vasoconstriction and coagulation.

a. Vasoconstriction: Immediately after injury, there is constriction of injured vessels to prevent excessive blood loss. This vasoconstriction lasts for 5–10 minutes.

b. Coagulation: There is clot formation with the help of fibrin and platelets; the coagulation cascade activates fibrin deposition and strengthens the clot.

During this phase, platelets release growth factors like platelet-derived growth factor (PDGF) and transforming growth factor-beta (TGF-β), which in turn are responsible for initiating the healing cascade.

2.2 Inflammatory phase (1st to 6th day)

It includes the following processes [3–5]:

a. Vasodilation and increased capillary permeability: This is mediated with the help of histamine, serotonin (released by platelets), and nitrous oxide (released by endothelial cells).

b. Chemotaxis: This is initiated by the release of alpha granule products within platelet cells, complement activation factor (C5a), coagulation cascade factors, and tissue products, as well as some bacterial products.

c. Cell migration

- The blood cells get adherent to the vessel wall (margination), then they traverse through the vessel wall (diapedesis) into the extravascular matrix, which is initially composed mostly of fibrin.

d. Cellular response

- Neutrophils (appear from 24 to 48 hours): They are the first responders, engulfing pathogens and debris by phagocytosis. However, in conditions where neutrophils are absent, the wound healing process remains unaffected.

- Macrophages (appear from 48 to 96 hours): Macrophages replace neutrophils and release cytokines such as tumor necrosis factor-alpha (TNF-α) and interleukin-1 (IL-1), which promote fibroblast activation. The macrophages are very important for wound healing, as they produce important growth factors.

- Lymphocytes (appear from 5th to 7th day): They regulate collagenase and extracellular matrix (ECM) remodeling.

2.3 Fibro-proliferative phase (from 4th day to 3rd week)

This phase of healing comprises the following processes [3, 6]:

a. Matrix formation

- Fibroblasts: They start appearing in the wound from 2nd to 3rd day, and by 1 week, they become the most dominant cells in the wound; they start collagen deposition in the wound from 5th day to 3rd week. Granulation tissue, rich in fibroblasts and newly formed capillaries, replaces fibrin clots.

- Glycosaminoglycan (GAG) production: Initially, hyaluronic acid is produced, followed by chondroitin-4 sulfate, heparin sulfate, and dermatan sulfate, which is followed by collagen production.

- Tensile strength starts increasing from 4th to 5th day.

  i. Angiogenesis: Vascular endothelial growth factor (VEGF) and nitrous oxide production lead to an increase in vascularity from parent vessels.

  ii. Epithelialization: It consists of the following activities:

- Mobilization: Loss of contact inhibition; cells at the edge of the wound, as well as in skin appendages (in partial-thickness wounds), become flat and then break contact (integrin) with the neighboring cells.

- Migration: Cells move across the wound till they meet cells from the other end of the wound, and once they meet, the contact inhibition is re-established.

- Mitosis: The cells in the wound edges migrate to cover the wound gap, while the basal cells at the edge of the wound divide to produce a greater number of cells required for filling the wound gap.

- Differentiation: The new cells covering the wound re-establish all epithelial skin layers, from the lower basal layer to the top layer of stratum corneum, after migration is completed.

2.4 Remodeling/maturation phase (from 3rd week to 1 year)

- The collagen formation and its breakdown are balanced by 3–5 weeks of the wound healing process [3]. So, there is no net change in overall collagen quantity, but there is an increase in organization of collagen and strengthening of cross-links.

- Type III collagen is replaced by Type I collagen during the remodeling phase to restore the normal ratio of 4:1 between Type 1 and Type III collagen.

- Myofibroblasts facilitate wound contraction.

- Excess blood vessels undergo apoptosis as vascular density normalizes. The glycosaminoglycans (GAGs), water quantity, and number of cells decrease during this phase.

Once the wound is completely healed, it achieves a maximum tensile strength of 80% of its pre-injury status. This is achieved by the end of 2 months of the healing process.

Growth factor	Function
VEGF	Endothelial cell proliferation
FGF	Fibroblast chemotaxis; fibroblast and keratinocyte proliferation
EGF	Fibroblasts and keratinocyte division and migration
TGF-beta	Fibroblast proliferation and migration
PDGF	Fibroblast cell, endothelial cell, and smooth muscle cell proliferation

VEGF: vascular endothelial growth factor, EGF: epithelial growth factor, FGF: fibroblast growth factor, PDGF: platelet-derived growth factor, TGF-beta: transforming growth factor-beta.

Table 1.
Growth factors and their roles in the process of wound healing.

3. Collagen production

The collagen is composed of three helically woven polypeptide chains [3, 7]. These polypeptide chains are mostly composed of hydroxylysine and hydroxyproline amino acids. There are more than 20 collagen types, which vary in amino acid sequences from each other.

- Type I: This is most abundant in our body and constitutes 90% of total body collagen; this form is dominant in bone, skin, and tendon.

- Type II: It is mostly found in the corneal part of the eye as well as in the hyaline type of cartilage.

- Type III: It is present in blood vessel walls, dermal skin, and uterine and gut walls.

- Type IV: It is found in the basement membrane.

4. Growth factors

The growth factors involved in the process of wound healing, along with their roles, are given in **Table 1** [3, 8–10].

5. Wound contraction

Myofibroblasts play a major role in wound contraction. These are specialized fibroblast cells and have contractile cytoplasmic microfilaments and distinct cellular adhesion structures (maculae adherens and desmosomes). They are dispersed widely in granulating wounds; they act synergistically in contracting the wound bed. By the 3rd day, the myofibroblasts appear in the wound, and by 10–21 days, they reach their optimal number. Myofibroblasts disappear as wound contraction is completed [3].

The thickness of the dermis in the wound determines the level of contraction that the wound undergoes; the more the dermis thickness in the wound, the lesser the extent of contraction it undergoes. This is the reason for less contraction in wounds covered by full-thickness skin grafts as compared to wounds covered by split-thickness skin grafts [8, 11].

6. Types of wound healing

There are three main mechanisms by which wounds can heal, which are governed by the type of wound and whether or not any intervention of wound approximation is performed [3].

i. Primary intention: Clean wounds like surgical incisions, which are closed within hours of creation by re-approximating edges. The granulation tissue formation is very minimal, and such wounds heal with minimal scarring.

ii. Secondary intention: Wounds with extensive tissue loss, such as pressure ulcers and burns, can heal by granulation tissue formation, contraction, and epithelialization. These wounds have a higher risk of infection and heal with excessive scar formation.

iii. Tertiary intention (delayed primary closure): Wounds that are initially not closed and left open due to high infection risk or due to post-traumatic wound contamination. The subacute or chronic wound is converted to an acute wound by sharp debridement and then closed primarily; healing is comparable to primary closure.

7. Factors affecting wound healing

7.1 Genetic

- Age affects healing rate; healing is faster and better in infants and children because aging reduces fibroblast activity and collagen synthesis [3].

- Various genetic factors lead to predisposition for keloid and hypertrophic scar formation.

- Skin type: The Fitzpatrick skin type, skin thickness, elasticity, sebaceous quality, and part of the body involved (e.g., sternum, shoulder, and earlobe have high vulnerability to hypertrophic scarring or keloid scar formation).

- Hereditary conditions:

    - Progeria: There is a mutation in the Lamin A/C (LMNA) gene. Affected patients present with a large head, limited growth, narrow face, beaked nose, full-body alopecia, wrinkled skin, and atherosclerosis. Surgery is not recommended in progeria patients because of defective healing.

    - Ehlers-Danlos syndrome: This condition is characterized by abnormal collagen production, impaired collagen processing, and its structure. These patients have fragile skin, which bruises easily with hypermobile joints and vascular aneurysms. Surgery is not recommended in patients with Ehlers-Danlos syndrome due to defective healing.

- o Werner syndrome: The Werner syndrome (WRN) gene is mutated in Werner syndrome [12]. This condition is an autosomal recessive disorder. Affected persons present with thickened skin, graying of hair, cataracts, hoarse voice, diabetes mellitus, and atherosclerosis. Surgery is not usually recommended, except in severe functional impairment or life-threatening conditions.

- o Cutis laxa is one of the rare defective connective tissue conditions, in which there is impairment in extracellular matrix formation, especially the elastic fibers. This condition is characterized by hypermobility in the joints with loose, wrinkled skin. Surgical excision of redundant skin, like abdominoplasty (excision of redundant abdominal skin) and blepharoplasty (correction of eyelid skin laxity), has just short-lasting benefits, as the recurrence rate is high.

- o Pseudoxanthoma elasticum is a rare genetic disorder characterized by fragmented and calcified elastic fibers. These patients present with increased skin laxity, visual impairment, and skin papules, which are mostly yellow colored. A patient's redundant skin folds can be treated with surgical excision.

7.2 Systemic health conditions

Systemic health conditions that affect healing are comorbidities, like [13].

- Immunodeficiency
- Diabetes
- Atherosclerotic disease
- Nutritional deficiencies
- Renal failure

7.3 Vitamins and minerals

- Vitamin A: It can reverse the delayed wound healing effect of steroids but cannot correct immunosuppression [14]. An oral dose of 25,000 IU daily increases tensile strength, or it can be applied topically, 200,000 IU every 8 hours, which can enhance wound epithelialization.

- Vitamin C: It acts as a cofactor for key enzymes involved in the hydroxylation of proline and lysine, which in turn are responsible for cross-linkage and strengthening of collagen. Deficiency of vitamin C leads to scurvy, which is characterized by decreased tensile strength, decreased collagen synthesis, capillary hemorrhage, and immature fibroblasts.

- Vitamin E: It helps in cell membrane stabilization and has the role of an antioxidant. But there can be impaired wound healing if high doses of vitamin E are consumed. There is no scientific evidence that it helps in reducing scar formation, and in turn, its excessive doses can cause dermatitis.

- Zinc: It acts as a cofactor for enzymes. Deficiency causes impaired fibroblast proliferation and epithelialization [3].

7.4 Drugs

Steroids affect wound healing by:

- Inhibiting epithelialization
- Decreasing inflammation
- Decreasing production of collagen

Antineoplastic agents

- These drugs affect rapidly dividing cells, which in the wound include keratinocytes, endothelial cells, and fibroblasts [15].
- Adverse effects of antineoplastic drugs on wound healing can be minimized by delaying their administration by 10–14 days after closure of the wound.

Anti-inflammatory medicines: They may affect healing by decreasing collagen synthesis.

Lathyrogens: These act by inhibiting the enzyme lysyl oxidase, which in turn causes impairment in wound healing. Lysyl oxidase enzyme impairment results in poor tensile strength, as it is responsible for cross-linking collagen fibrils. The known lathyrogens are beta-aminopropionitrile (BAPN), lathyrus plant legumes, and d-penicillamine.

Smoking: The cigarettes contain nicotine, which increases platelet adherence and clot formation, in addition to blood vessel constriction. The smoke contains carbon monoxide, which causes a reduction in oxygen delivery to body tissues.

7.5 Local wound factors

- Infection:

Wound infection affects healing by decreasing epithelialization, angiogenesis, and oxygen tension; lowering pH; and increasing collagenase activity.

- Tissue oxygenation:

One of the most common causes of failure of wound healing is poor blood supply and oxygen delivery to healing tissue, like in scleroderma, atherosclerosis, and Raynaud's disease. Angiogenesis is induced by the application of hyperbaric oxygen therapy in hypoxic wounds.

- Radiation therapy:

It damages the nuclei of growing cells and occludes small blood vessels, and hence leads to poor healing.

- Free radicals:

These impair wound healing due to an increase in reactive oxygen free radicals.

- Moisture balance:

Optimal hydration promotes epithelialization, while excessive moisture leads to maceration.

- Warmth:

Perfusion is increased by keeping wounds warm, which in turn helps in increasing the tensile strength of the healing wound.

- Foreign bodies:

They can serve as a nidus of infection and lead to a delay in the healing process.

- Chronic wound:

Chronic wounds have a high concentration of metalloproteases, which slow down healing. Once the chronic wounds undergo debridement, it removes excessive metalloproteases from the wound, turning the chronic wound into an acute wound state [3].

8. Scarring

Hypertrophic scars (HTS) (**Figure 1**) [3].

They are constituted of extracellular matrix, myofibroblast cells, and type III collagen, running parallel to the surface of the epidermis. In addition, it consists of abundant extracellular matrix and myofibroblast cells. A hypertrophic scar grows above the normal skin surface but does not breach the extent of the original wound. HTS are more common than keloid scars. Wounds that heal under tension and are located over flexor aspects of the body have a high predisposition for hypertrophic scar formation. Chances of recurrence are less in HTS post excision and adjuvant therapies as compared to keloid scars [16].

Keloid scars (**Figures 2** and **3**).

The term "Keloid" has been derived from a Greek word "Chele," which means claws of a crab [17]. Keloid scars typically extend beyond the original wound margins. They consist mostly of hypocellular matrix with disorganized type III and I collagen fibrils. Keloid scars are rare in newborns and the elderly and are seen only in human beings [3, 17].

Development of keloid scars is governed by genetic factors and is affected by body hormones, which make keloid formation more common during pregnancy and adolescence.

Keloid scars are very unlikely to regress on their own, and there is a high rate of recurrence post any treatment, including excision; therefore, multimodality treatment methods are recommended for the management of keloid scars [18].

DOI: http://dx.doi.org/10.5772/intechopen.1012688

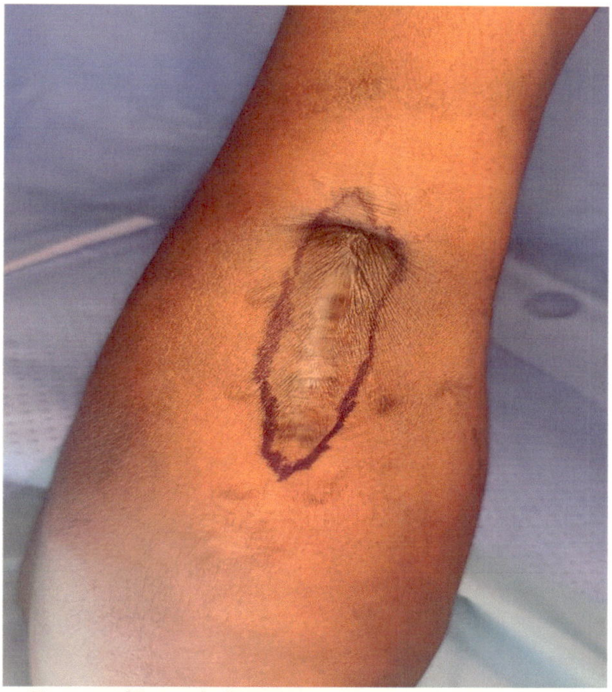

Figure 1.
Hypertrophic scar in forearm.

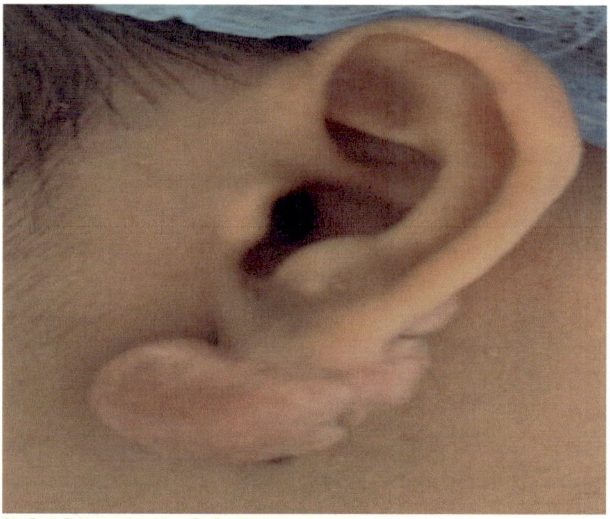

Figure 2.
Keloid scar in ear lobule.

Scar management [19–22].

- Excision: Removal of scar tissue is one of the most successful methods for treating scars, with a success rate in preventing recurrence ranging from 50 to 100%.

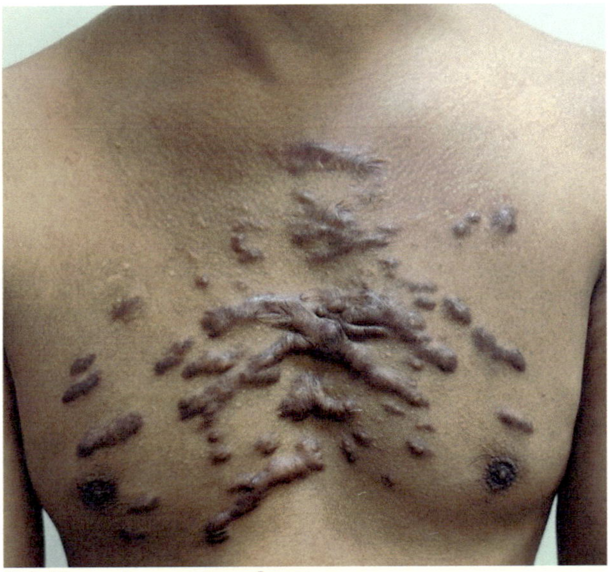
Keloid scar in pre-sternal area

Figure 3.
Keloid scar in presternal area.

- Radiation: It inhibits angiogenesis and fibroblast proliferation, with a recurrence rate of keloid scar postradiation therapy ranging from 2 to 33%.

- Corticosteroids: Their mechanism of action for treating keloids and HTS is through reduction in inflammation and collagen synthesis. However, post corticosteroid treatment, recurrence can be observed in as many as half of the treated patients. Potential risks of steroid infiltration into a scar include telangiectasia, subcutaneous atrophy, and skin hypopigmentation.

- 5-Fluorouracil (5-FU): Fibroblast proliferation is inhibited by 5-FU. The recurrence rate of around 19% has been reported post-5-FU treatment of keloid scars.

- Interferon: They act by reducing the production of fibroblasts and glycosaminoglycans and by increasing collagenase activity. The post-interferon treatment recurrence rate of keloid scars is about 54%.

- Cryotherapy: It is helpful in the treatment of scars by modifying fibroblast differentiation and collagen synthesis. The recurrence rate of keloid scars post-treatment is as high as 80%, so cryotherapy is recommended as adjuvant therapy rather than a sole treatment entity in treating keloid scars.

- Silicone sheets: These increase temperature and collagenase activity and help in the moisturization of the scar. It can be used as a preventive measure. Silicone sheet application is recommended as soon as wound epithelialization is complete and continued for at least a month [3].

- Scar massaging and pressure therapy: They help in reducing scar thickness.

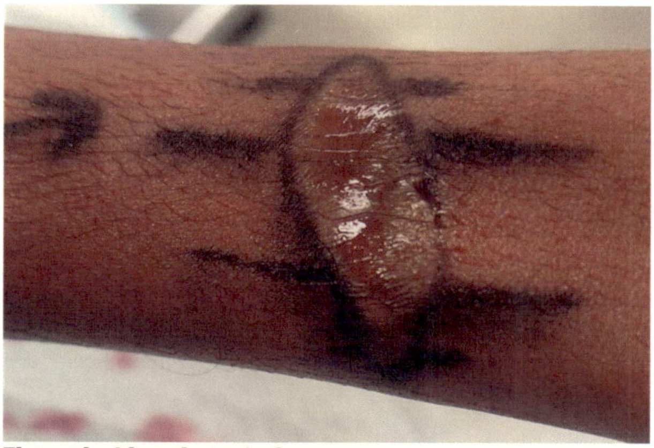

Flat and widened scar in forearm

Figure 4.
Flat and widened scar in forearm.

Widened scars (**Figure 4**).

Wide and depressed scars usually arise if the wound is under tension during healing and if there is increased mobility of the scar during its maturation phase.

9. Fetal wound healing

During the first two trimesters, the fetus has the potential for scarless healing. Fetal wound healing occurs without an inflammatory phase and without any angiogenesis. A high concentration of type III collagen and hyaluronic acid is found in the fetal wounds [3].

10. Clinical wound management

The management of any wound depends upon various factors, like whether the wound is clean or contaminated, acute or chronic, and surgical or traumatic. The management of surgically closed incisions is very different from non-healing wounds [8]. The management of some wound types is given below:

10.1 Incisional wounds

Incisional wounds are closed in layers and heal by primary intention. Deep sutures are placed in fascia or dermis, which can hold wound edges together even under high tension [23]. Fatty tissue layers do not need to be sutured, as they cannot withstand any tension. Dead space on wound closure is managed by placement of a closed suction drain for a brief period postoperatively, thereby preventing seroma formation and any infection. The small, clean wounds that are closed heal faster with minimal scar formation, whereas large, open, dirty wounds heal slowly and can result in excessive scar formation. To prevent hematoma formation, meticulous hemostasis needs to be achieved, which otherwise can serve as a nidus for infection and subsequent excessive scar formation.

The width of scars can be minimized by meticulous approximation of wound edges, avoiding any skin edge injury by meticulous handling of tissues. The suture material acts as a foreign body and can induce a foreign body reaction, which in turn might result in inflammation as well as infection of the sutured wound [24]. So, the use of fibrin glues and sealants, especially in superficial wounds in infants, can decrease scar formation [25].

Closed wounds take around 24–48 hours for epithelization, and after that, the patient can be allowed to take a shower or wash. In closed incisional wounds, tensile strength of 20% is achieved at 3 weeks, and 70% on completion of 6 weeks of healing [23]. The maximum tensile strength that is achieved after complete wound healing is around 75–80% of that of normal skin tensile strength. Therefore, if absorbable sutures are used for closure of wounds under tension, the suture should hold tensile strength for a minimum period of 6 weeks. So, it is advisable to avoid any heavy activity for around one and a half months of the postoperative period.

10.2 Excisional wounds

Open wounds as well as closed wounds heal through the same phases of inflammation, proliferation, and remodeling. But the main difference is the long time taken by each phase, especially the proliferative phase. There is a greater amount of granulation tissue formation and contraction, as it heals by secondary intention. Open wound edges are separated; thus, epithelial cells must move long distances. The infection, with high protein exudate, dysregulates healing and transforms the healing wound into a non-healing wound [23, 24].

A large-sized, well-granulated wound, which can delay healing by more than 2–3 weeks, should be covered either by a full-thickness or split-thickness skin graft. The split-thickness skin graft donor site takes around 14–21 days to heal, which mostly depends on the dermal thickness of the harvested skin graft. An open wound can easily break under stretching force as it heals by secondary intention and thereby has less tensile strength [26].

10.3 Wound treatment

Necrotic material should be debrided from open wounds, as it serves otherwise as a culture source for bacteria; the exception to immediate debridement is a dry eschar without any evidence of infection. Open wounds need a moist and sterile environment to heal [27, 28].

10.3.1 Chronic open wounds

A team approach is required for the optimal management of chronic wounds, which includes a plastic surgeon, endocrinologist, microbiologist, vascular surgeon, orthopedic surgeon, podiatrist, and internist [23]. After debridement of necrotic tissue, wound moisture imbalances should be managed by proper dressing and compression therapy [29].

Associated comorbidities should be aggressively managed. The wound depth, size, infection, and edema should be documented, and local wound care is continued until the wound is ready for the reconstruction procedure or heals by secondary intention.

10.4 Wound dressings

Various wound dressings are available for different types of wounds [30]. Engineered skin replacements are of significant help in managing chronic wounds.

The ideal open wound dressing should maintain a moist, clean environment, stimulate repair, reduce edema, and not be expensive. Dressing changes should be done less frequently in clean wounds to enhance healing and prevent any skin irritation.

Wound dressings are classified according to their action (like debriding, absorbing, occlusive, antibacterial, adherence), the physical composition of the dressing (foam, gel, ointment, film), and the type of dressing material (e.g., hydrocolloid, collagen, alginate) (**Table 2**).

10.4.1 Film dressing

The films are gas-permeable dressings, maintain wound hydration, and are good for dressing partial-thickness dermal wounds like the skin graft donor site.

For wounds with high output exudate, the absorptive dressings are used to maintain a moist environment but without excessive fluid accumulation [24]. Hydrocolloid dressings are thick and can cover exudative wounds for almost 2–3 days, as their limit of absorptive capacity is reached; they lose adhesiveness and can be replaced with ease [32]. Alginates can absorb 15–20 times their weight and are hence used for high-exuding wounds [33].

Hydrogels have little adhesiveness and are useful for dressing facial wounds, ligaments, or tendons [34].

10.4.2 Vacuum-assisted closure

A vacuum-assisted closure (VAC) can be used on both inpatient and outpatient bases. A vacuum pump, sponge, and transparent film are required for the VAC application. Vacuum-assisted closure is useful to aid in the healing of venous stasis ulcers [35, 36], pressure ulcers, diabetic foot ulcers, complex leg ulcers, open abdominal wounds, traumatic wounds, and dehiscent sternal wounds [37]. Negative pressure in VAC can induce granulation tissue formation over exposed bones and tendons. VAC decreases tissue edema and bacterial wound colonization and, in addition, increases granulation tissue formation as well as increases local blood flow [38]. Mechanical forces by VAC deform tissues, which leads to stimulation of growth factor pathways and thereby increases production of new tissue [39, 40].

10.4.3 Compression therapy

Wound and edema in the lower extremity due to lymphedema, venous insufficiency, or cardiovascular disease should be treated by compression therapy and limb elevation. Four-layer dressing wraps are commonly used in lower extremity edema. Once the venous stasis wound heals, it is recommended to continuously wear the pressure stocking of pressure 30–40 mmHg [41]. Compression dressing should be applied with caution in patients with peripheral neuropathy and arteriosclerosis. Intermittent compression therapy through an electrically inflatable boot applying pressure ranging from 20 to 120 mm Hg can be helpful adjuvant therapy in lymphedema associated with chronic leg ulcers [42].

10.4.4 Pharmacologic treatment

Pharmacological agents like collagenases (streptokinase, streptodornase) are used for debridement of thin, superficial necrotic tissues on a minimal scale. However,

Class	Composition	Characteristics and function	Commercial examples
Absorptive powder and paste	Starch copolymers, hydrocolloid particles	Can be used as filler in deep wounds; high exudate absorption capacity	Aquacel, Granugel paste, Geliperm, Duoderm granules
Gauze	Consists of woven fibers of cotton	Permeable to water; for wound debridement (wet-to-dry dressing); removal from the wound is painful	Curity, Mepitel, Mepilex
Tulles	Soft paraffin or iodine or chlorhexidine-impregnated open-weave fiber dressing	Non-adherent, hydrophobic dressing. suitable for shallow wounds with less exudation	Adaptic, Jelonet, Tullegras, Urgotul
Film	Semipermeable; plastic (polyurethane)	Adhesive dressing; impermeable to liquids and bacteria but allows water vaporization	Opsite, Tegaderm
Foam	Semipermeable; silicone or polyurethane foams with outer surface (hydrophobic) and inner wound surface (hydrophilic)	High absorbing capacity; used for exudative and necrotic wounds	Tielle, Allevyn, Lyofoam
Hydrogel	Water (96%) and polymer (polyethylene oxide)	Aqueous environment; requires secondary dressing; no adherence; not recommended if infection is present; semipermeable	Aquaform, Intrasite, Purilon, Vigilon, Aquasorb
Hydrocolloid	Adhesive hydrophilic colloidal particles	Occlusive dressing; absorbs fluid; necrotic tissue autolysis; little adherence	Intrasite, Comfeel, Tegasorb, Duoderm
Alginate	Calcium and sodium salts of alginic acid are found in brown seaweed	High exudate absorption capacity; forms a hydrophilic gel after an ion exchange with the fluid in the wound; not advisable for dry wounds	Sorbsan, Algisite, Algosteril, Kaltostat SeaSorb, Suprasorb
Antimicrobial dressings	1. Silver (in ionic or nanocrystalline form) 2. Iodine a. as povidone-iodine b. as cadexomer iodine 3. Metronidazole gel 4. Octinidine gel	Suited for colonized or infected wounds: 1. Absorptive: cadexomer iodine (caution: thyroid diseases) 2. In fungating malignant wounds, they control odor by inhibiting the growth of anaerobic bacteria 3. Used for burns	1. Acticoat, Actisorb, Silver 200, Aquacel Ag 2. Iodosorb 3. Metrotop Gel 4. Octinidine/Lavanid Gel
Silicone	Silicone sheets	Increases skin temperature, sheet induces a localized electromagnetic field, and decreases scar formation	Mepilex, Sil-K, Mepitel

Class	Composition	Characteristics and function	Commercial examples
Sub-atmospheric pressure	Vacuum pump, sponge, plastic film	Sponge conforms to the wound, and vacuum removes edema fluid and bacteria; stimulation of granulation, vascularization, and wound cell proliferation	VAC device
Dermal collagen replacement	Porcine dermal collagen with fine fibric mesh fabric (nylon, silicone)	Non-adherent; Semipermeable	Biobrane
Dermal matrix replacement	Acellular matrix	Stimulates repair; Permeable	Integra (composed of silicone sheet, shark cartilage, and bovine collagen); AlloDerm (human, dermis); SIS (porcine, small-bowel submucosa),
Dermal living replacement	Absorbable matrix populated with allogenic human fibroblasts	Permeable; increased stimulation of repair	Dermagraft (bioabsorbable scaffold); TransCyte (nylon mesh coated with porcine collagen)
Epidermal living replacement	Autologous keratinocytes cultured on murine feeder cells	Permeable; increased stimulation of repair	Epicel
Skin living replacement	Bovine collagen matrix populated with neonatal human fibroblasts with an outer layer of human keratinocytes	Impermeable; increased stimulation of repair	Apligraf, OrCel
Amnion/chorion allograft	Human placental derivatives Human amnion/chorion	Modulates inflammation, enhances healing, and reduces excessive scar formation	Epifix, Amniofix

Table 2.
Different wound dressings, their composition, and characteristics [3, 23, 31].

collagenase can be detrimental to a clean wound in the proliferative phase; hence, it should be avoided in healing wounds [24].

10.4.5 Skin substitutes

With the help of tissue engineering technology, various skin and dermal substitutes have been made available. They have the additional benefit of accelerating wound healing because of the presence of growth factors [23]. These skin substitutes are placed on open wounds like autologous skin grafts with bolster dressing support [43]. The skin substitutes have the advantage of being able to cover large wounds when there are inadequate skin donor sites available, they can be applied bedside, and there is no donor site morbidity. Some skin substitute disadvantages are limited shelf life, high price, and they are not easily available [44]. The bi-layered human keratinocyte-fibroblast construct on a bovine collagen matrix is called Apligraf, which is a bi-layered human keratinocyte-fibroblast with bovine collagen matrix. It improves healing in diabetic wounds, venous stasis wounds, and arterial insufficiency wounds [45–47].

Cultured epidermal autograft (Epicel) takes 2–3 weeks to get ready through the culture process and is used for treating second- and third-degree burns [48]. In addition to a long culture time disadvantage, they are difficult to handle and may lead to blistering [49].

10.4.6 Amnion/chorion membrane allograft

These are composed of a bioactive tissue matrix containing human chorion/amnion membrane constituents. It consists of an extracellular matrix (collagen, elastin, and proteoglycans) with various growth factors. They enhance healing, reduce inflammation, and overall scar formation [50].

11. Future perspectives

11.1 Growth factors

Various growth factors, FGF, PDGF, and TGF-β, have been studied for use in chronic and burn wounds [51]. GM-CSF has shown good efficacy in venous leg ulcers. Topical recombinant bovine FGF and human KGF (Repifermin) have been found effective in chronic pressure ulcers, and granulocyte colony-stimulating factor and TGF-β2 were effective in diabetic foot ulcers [52]. However, so far only PDGF-BB has been licensed for commercial use in the US and Europe for chronic wound therapy [23]. Challenges in the use of growth factors for wound therapy are increased protease activity in chronic wounds, cost, and the development of specific antibodies against growth factors [34, 42, 53–56].

11.2 Gene therapy

Gene therapy is the introduction of a growth factor gene or other therapeutic gene into growing wound cells to enhance the healing process. Once the gene is introduced into the cell, its expression is sustained at a therapeutic level; its expression is stopped when it is no longer needed. Various gene delivery vehicles are being developed, like retrovirus, replication-deficient adenovirus, and herpes simplex virus type 1 [57]. Other non-viral delivery approaches are physical and chemical gene transfer using liposomes. IGF-1, KGF, FGF, and VEGF genes have been transferred into wound cells [58–61]. In some experimental studies, direct injection of genes using a gene gun has been used for EGF, TGF-β1, and PDGF gene transfer into the wounds [62–64]. The safety, feasibility, and biologic plausibility are being tested in a phase I clinical trial of adenovirus-mediated rhPDGF-BB gene treatment of venous leg ulcers [65].

11.3 Stem cell therapy

Multipotent adult stem cells are easily accessible and are available in abundance for the treatment of chronic wounds. Mesenchymal stem cells (MSCs) and epidermal stem cells are currently available for use in adults [66]. Epidermal stem cells present in the basal layer of skin and hair follicles contribute to re-epithelialization of chronic wounds [67, 68]. MSCs can trans-differentiate into tissues of mesodermal origin, e.g., bone, fat, skeletal muscle, cartilage, and tendons, or they can "cross-differentiate" into other non-mesodermal cells [69–71]. Bone marrow-derived MSCs and adipose tissue-derived mesenchymal stem cells (adMSCs) are being studied for use in chronic wounds [72, 73].

12. Conclusion

Wound healing is a complex and dynamic process. Effective wound management requires a thorough understanding of the distinct phases of wound healing as well as factors that affect wound healing. Advances in wound care technologies have revolutionized the treatment approach, offering improved outcomes for acute and chronic wounds.

However, challenges still exist, especially in the management of non-healing wounds in patients with comorbidities. A patient-centered approach incorporating evidence-based practices is essential for optimizing healing and preventing complications. Future research should explore new therapies to enhance wound healing and tissue regeneration.

Acknowledgements

Open access funding provided by Qatar National Library.

Conflict of interest

The author declares no conflict of interest.

Thanks, note

I want to express my deepest gratitude and thanks to our Hamad Medical Corporation Plastic Surgery section head, Dr. Atalla Hammouda, for his continuous, unwavering support and encouragement.

Author details

Tawheed Ahmad
Hamad Medical Corporation, Qatar

*Address all correspondence to: drtawheedahmad@yahoo.com

References

[1] Trace AP, Enos CW, Mantel A, et al. Keloids and hypertrophic scars: A Spectrum of clinical challenges. American Journal of Clinical Dermatology. 2016;**17**:201-223. DOI: 10.1007/s40257-016-0175-7

[2] Cho YD, Kim KH, Lee YM, Ku Y, Seol YJ. Periodontal wound healing and tissue regeneration: A narrative review. Pharmaceuticals (Basel). 2021;**14**(5):456. DOI: 10.3390/ph14050456

[3] Parker TH 3rd, Harrison B. Wound healing. In: Janis JE, editor. Essentials of Plastic Surgery. 2nd ed. Boca Raton: CRC Press; 2014. p. 7. eBook ISBN: 9780429173196

[4] Pang C, Ibrahim A, Bulstrode NW, Ferretti P. An overview of the therapeutic potential of regenerative medicine in cutaneous wound healing. International Wound Journal. 2017 Jun;**14**(3):450-459. DOI: 10.1111/iwj.12735. Epub 2017 Mar 6

[5] Peterson CY, Shaterian A, Borboa AK, Gonzalez AM, Potenza BM, Coimbra R, et al. The noninvasive, quantitative, in vivo assessment of adenoviral-mediated gene delivery in skin wound biomaterials. Biomaterials. 2009;**30**(35):6788-6793. DOI: 10.1016/j.biomaterials.2009.07.069

[6] Ather S, Harding KG. Wound management and dressings. In: Rajendran S, editor. Advanced Textiles for Wound Care. Cambridge: Woodhead Publishing; 2009. pp. 3-19. DOI: 10.1533/9781845696306.1.3. ISBN: 9781845692711

[7] Stadelmann WK, Digenis AG, Tobin GR. Physiology and healing dynamics of chronic cutaneous wounds. American Journal of Surgery. 1998;**176**(Suppl. 2):26S-38S

[8] Herndon DN. Total Burn Care. 3rd ed. Edinburgh: Saunders Elsevier; 2007. ISBN 978-1-4160-3274-8

[9] Hade MD, Suire CN, Mossell J, Suo Z. Extracellular vesicles: Emerging frontiers in wound healing. Medicinal Research Reviews. 2022;**42**(4):21918. DOI: 10.1002/med.21918

[10] Majnooni MB, Fakhri S, Smeriglio A, Trombetta D, Croley CR, Bhattacharyya P, et al. Antiangiogenic effects of coumarins against cancer: From chemistry to medicine. Molecules. 2019;**24**(23):4278. DOI: 10.3390/molecules24234278

[11] James MI. Alteration of split skin graft contraction with a synthetic dressing. European Journal of Plastic Surgery. 1990;**13**:97-100. DOI: 10.1007/BF00170317

[12] Lee JH, Shamanna RA, Kulikowicz T, Borhan Fakouri N, Kim EW, Christiansen LS, et al. CDK2 phosphorylation of Werner protein (WRN) contributes to WRN's DNA double-strand break repair pathway choice. Aging Cell. 2021;**20**(11):e13484. DOI: 10.1111/acel.13484. Epub 2021 Oct 6

[13] Janis JE, Kwon RK, Lalonde DH. A practical guide to wound healing. Plastic and Reconstructive Surgery. 2010;**125**:230e-244e

[14] Janis JE, Harrison B. Wound healing: Part I. Basic science. Plastic and Reconstructive Surgery. 2014;**133**(2):199e-207e. DOI: 10.1097/01.prs.0000437224.02985.f9

[15] Falcone RE, Nappi JF. Chemotherapy and wound healing. The Surgical Clinics of North America. 1984;**64**:779-794

[16] Khoo TL, Halim AS, Saad AZM, Dorai AA, Jaafar H. A prospective, randomised, double-blinded trial to study the efficacy of topical tocotrienol in the prevention of hypertrophic scars. Journal of Plastic, Reconstructive & Aesthetic Surgery. 2011;**64**(6):e137-e145. DOI: 10.1016/j.bjps.2011.02.004

[17] Seo BF, Lee JY, Jung SN. Models of abnormal scarring. BioMed Research International. 2013;**2013**:423147. DOI: 10.1155/2013/423147. Epub 2013 Sep 3

[18] Chike-Obi CJ, Cole PD, Brissett AE. Keloids: Pathogenesis, clinical features, and management. Seminars in Plastic Surgery. 2009;**23**:178-184

[19] Mustoe TA, Cooter RD, Gold MH, et al. International clinical recommendations on scar management. Plastic and Reconstructive Surgery. 2002;**110**:560-571

[20] Shin TM, Bordeaux JS. The role of massage in scar management: A literature review. Dermatologic Surgery. 2012;**38**:414-423

[21] Khoo TL, Halim AS, Zakaria Z, et al. A prospective, randomized, double-blinded trial to study the efficacy of topical tocotrienol in the prevention of hypertrophic scars. Journal of Plastic, Reconstructive & Aesthetic Surgery. 2011;**64**:e137-e145

[22] Chung VQ, Kelley L, Marra D, et al. Onion extract gel versus petrolatum emollient on new surgical scars: Prospective double-blinded study. Dermatologic Surgery. 2006;**32**:193-219

[23] Mirastschijski U, Jokuszies A, Vogt P. Skin Wound Healing: Repair Biology, Wound and Scar Treatment. Philadelphia, PA: Elsevier Saunders; 2012

[24] Lorenz HP, Longaker MT. Wounds: Biology, pathology, and management. In: Norton JA et al., editors. Surgery. New York, NY: Springer; 2008. DOI: 10.1007/978-0-387-68113-9_10

[25] Vogt PM, Altintas MA, Radtke C, et al. Bases and methods of suturing. Der Chirurg. 2009;**80**(437-444):446-447

[26] Plá Sánchez F, Rial R, Cernuda Artero I, Ruíz Álvarez P, Moñux Ducajú G, Martínez López I, et al. Free skin micrografts with cyanoacrylate as outpatient treatment for venous leg ulcers. Journal of Wound Care. 2019;**28**(10):670-675. DOI: 10.12968/jowc.2019.28.10.670

[27] Vogt PM, Andree C, Breuing K, et al. Dry, moist, and wet skin wound repair. Annals of Plastic Surgery. 1995;**34**:493-499; discussion 499-500

[28] Svensjo T, Pomahac B, Yao F, et al. Accelerated healing of full-thickness skin wounds in a wet environment. Plastic and Reconstructive Surgery. 2000;**106**:602-612; discussion 613-4

[29] Schultz GS, Sibbald RG, Falanga V, et al. Wound bed preparation: A systematic approach to wound management. Wound Repair and Regeneration. 2003;**11**(Suppl 1):S1-S28

[30] Chaby G, Senet P, Vaneau M, et al. Dressings for acute and chronic wounds: A systematic review. Archives of Dermatology. 2007;**143**:1297-1304

[31] Jones V, Grey JE, Harding KG. Wound dressings. BMJ. 2006;**332**(7544):777-780. DOI: 10.1136/bmj.332.7544.777

[32] Norton JA, Bollinger RR, Chang AE, Lowry SF, Mulvihill SJ, Pass HI, et al. Surgery: Basic Science and Clinical Evidence. 1st ed. Berlin, Heidelberg: Springer; 2001. 2170 p

[33] Haxho F, Lytvyn Y, Shelley AJ, Ortega A, Melin M, Alavi A. Wound Care - Part I: A practical approach to local wound care and dressing selection. Journal of the American Academy of Dermatology. 20 Jun 2025:S0190-9622(25)02374-6. DOI: 10.1016/j.jaad.2025.02.103 [Epub ahead of print]

[34] Jones V, Grey JE, Harding KG. Wound dressings. BMJ. 2006;**332**:777-780

[35] Argenta LC, Morykwas MJ. Vacuum-assisted closure: A new method for wound control and treatment: Clinical experience. Annals of Plastic Surgery. 1997;**38**:563-576; discussion 577

[36] Genecov DG, Schneider AM, Morykwas MJ, et al. A controlled subatmospheric pressure dressing increases the rate of skin graft donor site reepithelialization. Annals of Plastic Surgery. 1998;**40**:219-225

[37] Apelqvist J, Armstrong DG, Augustin M, et al. Vacuum assisted closure: Recommendations for use. A consensus document. International Wound Journal. 2008;**5**(Suppl. 4):iii-19

[38] Morykwas MJ, Simpson J, Punger K, et al. Vacuum-assisted closure: State of basic research and physiologic foundation. Plastic and Reconstructive Surgery. 2006;**117**(Suppl.):121S-126S

[39] Silver FH, Siperko LM, Seehra GP. Mechanobiology of force transduction in dermal tissue. Skin Research and Technology. 2003;**9**:3-23

[40] Venturi ML, Attinger CE, Mesbahi AN, et al. Mechanisms and clinical applications of the vacuum-assisted closure (VAC) device: A review. American Journal of Clinical Dermatology. 2005;**6**:185-194

[41] Falanga V. Care of venous leg ulcers. Ostomy/Wound Management. 1999;**45**(Suppl. 1A):33S-43S; quiz 44S-45S

[42] Enoch S, Grey JE, Harding KG. ABC of wound healing. Non-surgical and drug treatments. BMJ. 2006;**332**:900-903

[43] Falanga V, Sabolinski M. A bilayered living skin construct (APLIGRAF) accelerates complete closure of hard-to-heal venous ulcers. Wound Repair and Regeneration. 1999;**7**:201-207

[44] Schonfeld WH, Villa KF, Fastenau JM, et al. An economic assessment of Apligraf (Graftskin) for the treatment of hard-to-heal venous leg ulcers. Wound Repair and Regeneration. 2000;**8**:251-257

[45] Ehrenreich M, Ruszczak Z. Update on tissue-engineered biological dressings. Tissue Engineering. 2006;**12**:2407-2424

[46] Mirastschijski U, Bugdahl R, Rollman O, et al. Epithelial regeneration from bioengineered skin explants in culture. The British Journal of Dermatology. 2006;**154**:42-49

[47] Falanga V, Isaacs C, Paquette D, et al. Wounding of bioengineered skin: Cellular and molecular aspects after injury. The Journal of Investigative Dermatology. 2002;**119**:653-660

[48] Ongarora BG. Recent technological advances in the management of chronic wounds: A literature review. Health Science Reports. 2022;**5**(3):e641. DOI: 10.1002/hsr2.641

[49] Macri L, Clark RA. Tissue engineering for cutaneous wounds: Selecting the proper time and space for growth factors, cells and the extracellular matrix. Skin Pharmacology and Physiology. 2009;**22**:83-93

[50] Koob TJ, Lim JJ, Massee M, Zabek N, Denozière G. Properties of dehydrated human amnion/chorion composite grafts: Implications for wound repair and soft tissue regeneration. Journal of Biomedial Materials Research Part B Applied Biomaterials. 2014;**2014**(102B):1353-1362

[51] Gohil S, James E, Nair L. Nanotechnologies to promote skin tissue regeneration. In: Laurencin CT, Nair LS, editors. Nanotechnology and Regenerative Engineering: The Scaffold. 2nd ed. Boca Raton: CRC Press; 2014. pp. 343-366. DOI: 10.1201/b17444-17. ISBN: 1466585382, 9781466585386

[52] Pastar I, Ojeh N, Glinos GD, Stojadinovic O, Tomic-Canic M. Physiology and pathophysiology of wound healing in diabetes. In: Veves A, Giurini JM, Guzman RJ, editors. The Diabetic Foot: Medical and Surgical Management. 4th ed. Cham: Humana; 2018. pp. 109-130. DOI: 10.1007/978-3-319-89869-8_8

[53] Yager DR, Nwomeh BC. The proteolytic environment of chronic wounds. Wound Repair and Regeneration. 1999;7:433-441

[54] Fray MJ, Dickinson RP, Huggins JP, et al. A potent, selective inhibitor of matrix metalloproteinase-3 for the topical treatment of chronic dermal ulcers. Journal of Medicinal Chemistry. 2003;**46**:3514-3525

[55] Makinen K, Manninen H, Hedman M, et al. Increased vascularity detected by digital subtraction angiography after VEGF gene transfer to human lower limb artery: A randomized, placebo-controlled, double-blinded phase II study. Molecular Therapy. 2002;**6**:127-133

[56] Steed DL. Clinical evaluation of recombinant human platelet-derived growth factor for the treatment of lower extremity diabetic ulcers. Diabetic ulcer study group. Journal of Vascular Surgery. 1995;**21**:71-78; discussion 79-81

[57] Hirsch T, Spielmann M, Yao F, et al. Gene therapy in cutaneous wound healing. Frontiers in Bioscience. 2007;**12**:2507-2518

[58] Vogt PM, Thompson S, Andree C, et al. Genetically modified keratinocytes transplanted to wounds reconstitute the epidermis. Proceedings of the National Academy of Sciences of the United States of America. 1994;**91**:9307-9311

[59] Sun L, Xu L, Chang H, et al. Transfection with aFGF cDNA improves wound healing. The Journal of Investigative Dermatology. 1997;**108**:313-318

[60] Jeschke MG, Richter G, Hofstadter F, et al. Non-viral liposomal keratinocyte growth factor (KGF) cDNA gene transfer improves dermal and epidermal regeneration through stimulation of epithelial and mesenchymal factors. Gene Therapy. 2002;**9**:1065-1074

[61] Taub PJ, Marmur JD, Zhang WX, et al. Locally administered vascular endothelial growth factor cDNA increases survival of ischemic experimental skin flaps. Plastic and Reconstructive Surgery. 1998;**102**:2033-2039

[62] Benn SI, Whitsitt JS, Broadley KN, et al. Particle-mediated gene transfer with transforming growth factor-beta1 cDNAs enhances wound repair in rat skin. The Journal of Clinical Investigation. 1996;**98**:2894-2902

[63] Andree C, Swain WF, Page CP, et al. In vivo transfer and expression of a human epidermal growth factor gene accelerates wound repair. Proceedings of the National Academy of Sciences

of the United States of America. 1994;**91**:12188-12192

[64] Eming SA, Whitsitt JS, He L, et al. Particle-mediated gene transfer of PDGF isoforms promotes wound repair. The Journal of Investigative Dermatology. 1999;**112**:297-302

[65] Margolis DJ, Morris LM, Papadopoulos M, et al. Phase I study of H5. 020CMV.PDGF-beta to treat venous leg ulcer disease. Molecular Therapy. 2009;**17**:1822-1829

[66] Akhter J, Aziz AA, Al AA. Stem cells and liver disease. Internet Journal of Medical Update. 2011 Jul;**6**(2):69-75. Available from: http://www.akspublication.com/ijmu

[67] Charruyer A, Ghadially R. Stem cells and tissue-engineered skin. Skin Pharmacology and Physiology. 2009;**22**:55-62

[68] Takahashi K, Tanabe K, Ohnuki M, et al. Induction of pluripotent stem cells from adult human fibroblasts by defined factors. Cell. 2007;**131**:861-872

[69] Schaffler A, Buchler C. Concise review: Adipose tissue-derived stromal cells–basic and clinical implications for novel cell-based therapies. Stem Cells. 2007;**25**:818-827

[70] Malgieri A, Kantzari E, Patrizi MP, Gambardella S. Bone marrow and umbilical cord blood human mesenchymal stem cells: State of the art. International Journal of Clinical and Experimental Medicine. 2010;**3**(4):248-269

[71] Badiavas EV, Falanga V. Treatment of chronic wounds with bone marrow-derived cells. Archives of Dermatology. 2003;**139**:510-516

[72] Bunnell BA, Flaat M, Gagliardi C, et al. Adipose-derived stem cells: Isolation, expansion and differentiation. Methods. 2008;**45**:115-120

[73] Duckers HJ, Pinkernell K, Milstein AM, et al. The bedside Celution system for isolation of adipose derived regenerative cells. EuroIntervention. 2006;**2**:395-398

Chapter 8

Hybrid Breast Reconstruction: Prepectoral Implant Combined with Lipofilling – Authors' Experience

Ioan-Constantin Pop, Maximilian-Vlad Muntean and Radu-Alexandru Ilies

Abstract

This chapter provides a comprehensive overview of hybrid breast reconstruction, an evolving technique that combines prepectoral implant placement with autologous lipofilling to enhance both aesthetic and functional outcomes in post-mastectomy patients. By positioning the implant above the pectoralis major muscle, this method aims to reduce postoperative pain, prevent muscle distortion, and maintain chest wall function. The addition of lipofilling improves soft tissue coverage, refines breast contour, and reduces implant visibility, particularly in thin patients, while also addressing common complications such as rippling. The chapter is structured to guide the reader through the broader oncologic context in which breast reconstruction is performed, including sections on the risk factors, pathogenesis, and genetics of breast cancer, as well as current screening and diagnostic methods. Treatment strategies are discussed with a focus on surgical management and reconstructive options. A brief overview of BIA-ALCL is included, given its relevance in implant-based reconstruction. The core sections detail the technical aspects of prepectoral reconstruction and describe the lipofilling technique as used by the author, drawing from clinical experience. Throughout, the chapter emphasizes surgical indications, patient selection, procedural nuances, and clinical outcomes, offering evidence-based insights and discussing both the benefits and limitations of this hybrid approach within contemporary breast reconstruction practices.

Keywords: breast reconstruction, breast cancer, prepectoral implant, fat grafting, polyurethane implant

1. Introduction

Breast cancer stands as a major global health challenge worldwide. It ranks as the most commonly diagnosed cancer worldwide, accounting for approximately 11.7% of all cancer cases. Among American women, breast cancer makes up

Category	Details
Protective Factors	Pregnancy, breastfeeding, regular exercise, healthy diet.
Modifiable Risk Factors	Obesity, poor dietary habits (e.g., chemical substances in food), alcohol, smoking, hormone therapy, exposure to ionizing radiation.
Genetic Risk Factors	5–10% of cases are hereditary, being caused by mutations in high-penetrance genes like BRCA1 and BRCA2.
Gene Function (BRCA1/2)	Tumor suppressor genes are involved in DNA repair. Mutations that occur reduce DNA repair capacity, increasing risk of developing cancer.
Genetic Risk Estimate	Lifetime risk for BRCA1/2 mutation carriers is estimated between 60 and 80%.
Other Genetic Insights	Low-penetrance variants contribute cumulatively to risk. Several gaps in knowledge still exist regarding the genetic predisposition.
High-Risk Management	Chemoprevention: Two FDA-approved drugs are used in high-risk patients. Prophylactic surgery is considered for mutation carriers.
Personalized Prevention	Requires precise individual risk estimation to optimize intervention strategies and minimize costs.

Table 1.
Overview of modifiable, genetic, and preventive aspects of breast cancer [3–6].

approximately 30% of all newly diagnosed cancers. Globally, it is the primary cause of cancer-related mortality among women [1]. Despite the higher incidence rates being reported in developed countries, a rising trend is observed in less developed regions. During the reproductive years, a significant upward trend is observed, followed by a slower rate of increase after the age of 50, the average age of menopause [2].

The diagnosis of breast cancer is established histologically using standardized pathological criteria. Invasive ductal carcinoma predominates among breast cancer histologies, comprising roughly half to three-quarters of all cases. In contrast, invasive lobular carcinoma is identified in 5–15% of patients, while combined and rare subtypes appear sporadically in clinical practice (**Table 1**) [7].

2. Risk factors, pathogenesis, and genetics of breast cancer

While multiple risk factors for breast cancer have been identified, the majority of cases, more than 75%, occur in women without any identifiable risk factors. Despite the higher rates observed in developed countries, the mortality in these areas is decreasing, due to the significant improvement in treatment protocols and the increased identification of the disease at an early stage. To reduce the treatment-related costs and social impact of breast cancer at the community level, prevention remains the most effective strategy. Both primary and secondary prevention play a crucial role [8]. Primary prevention aims to reduce cancer incidence by addressing extrinsic risk factors conditioned by lifestyle. Dietary habits are one of the most important risk factors. Excess weight and chemical substances found in food may promote neoplastic transformation in mammary gland cells [9]. Other preventive measures include: healthy diet, engaging in regular physical activity, and avoiding known risk factors such as tobacco use, excessive alcohol consumption, exogenous female hormones, and exposure to ionizing radiation. A protective effect against breast cancer has also been observed in women who have experienced pregnancy and engaged in breastfeeding [10]. For optimal personalized prevention, it is essential to accurately estimate a patient's breast cancer risk. This enables preventive interventions to be tailored to the individual's risk profile, leading to greater effectiveness and reduced costs. For high-risk patients, the U.S. Food and Drug Administration (FDA) has approved two chemoprevention medications, and in patients with genetic mutations, prophylactic surgery is recommended (**Table 2**) [8].

The etiology of breast cancer can be divided into genetic or non-genetic risk factors. About 5–10% of breast cancers are hereditary, caused by inherited genetic mutations that significantly increase the risk of developing the disease. Despite the evolution in this genetic domain, there are a lot of gaps. Despite advances in the field of cancer genetics, many knowledge gaps remain. Current understanding of breast cancer susceptibility indicates that a small subset of highly penetrant mutations (BRCA1 and BRCA2 genes) contributes significantly to risk. In addition, numerous genetic variants with lower penetrance collectively influence an individual's susceptibility. The interaction with other risk factors also plays an important role in the development of breast cancer. BRCA1 and BRCA2 are tumor suppressor genes that produce proteins that help repair damaged DNA and offer stability to cells. If a mutation occurs in these genes, the cells have a reduced ability to repair DNA, which increases the risk of developing cancer. Women carrying these mutations face a substantially increased lifetime risk of breast cancer, estimated between 60 and 80% (**Tables 3** and **4**) [11].

Pathogenic mechanism	Key factors/components	Explanation
Ductal hyperproliferation	Ductal epithelial cells	Initial stage, where an excessive proliferation can lead to benign or malignant tumors under persistent carcinogenic stimuli.
Tumor microenvironment (TME)	Stromal cells, macrophages, inflammatory mediators	Stroma alone could initiate tumorigenesis in experimental models; macrophages contribute to angiogenesis and immune evasion.
Inflammation & mutagenesis	Inflammatory cytokines, reactive species	Inflammation induces DNA damage and is responsible for a pro-tumorigenic environment.
Epigenetic modifications	DNA methylation	Distinct methylation patterns are seen in tumor vs. normal stroma and support the role of TME in promoting cancer.
Cancer stem cells (CSCs)	bCSCs, self-renewal pathways (Wnt, Notch, Hedgehog, PI3K, HIF, p53)	They represent a small population of therapy-resistant cells that initiate, maintain, and drive tumor recurrence. Their origin is most likely from the luminal progenitors.
Theoretical models of carcinogenesis	1. Cancer Stem Cell Theory 2. Stochastic Theory	CSC theory: All subtypes arise from mutated stem/progenitor cells. Stochastic theory: Any breast cell type might accumulate random mutations to become malignant.

Table 2.
Pathogenesis of breast cancer.

Category	Risk factor	Details/significance
Demographic	Aging	Incidence increases with age; 99.3% of deaths occur in women >40 years, 71.2% in women >60 years.
	Sex (female)	Female sex represents the most important non-modifiable risk factor.
Genetic/family	Family history	1st-degree relatives increase risk (1.75× for one, 2.5× for two or more).
	BRCA1/BRCA2 mutations	Strongly associated with hereditary breast cancer.
	Other genes	See below:
	– TP53	Mutations in 30% of breast cancers.
	– NME1	SNP linked to increased mortality and early-stage HR.
	– RB1	Inactivated in 20–35% of cases.
	– PTEN	Loss of expression in up to 33% of cases.
	– ATM	2–3x risk generally, 5–9x for women <50 years.
	– CDH1	Inactivated in 85% of lobular carcinomas.
	– FHIT	Hypermethylation 8.4× more frequent in cancer tissue.
	– Maspin	Expressed in 20–80% of invasive cases.
	– PIK3CA	Mutated in ~37% of HR+/HER2– metastatic & 40% early cancers.
	– CCND1 (Cyclin D1)	Overexpressed in ~50% of breast tumors.
Reproductive	Early menarche	Each year earlier increases risk by 5%.
	Late menopause	Each year delayed increases risk by 3%.
	Late first pregnancy (≥35 years)	HR = 1.54 compared to <20 years.
	Low parity	Risk decreases with more births (≥3 births: OR = 0.7 vs. nulliparae).
Hormonal	Endogenous estrogen	Ovariectomy reduces risk.
	Oral contraceptives	OR > 1.5 in African American and Iranian women; risk normalizes 10 years after stopping.
	Hormone replacement therapy (HRT)	RR = 1.66 in current users; HR = 1.95 after 8 years; recurrence HR = 3.6; risk decreases after 2 years of cessation.
Lifestyle/environment	Alcohol consumption	Each 10 g/day increases RR by 7.1%; 35–44 g/day → 32% increased risk.
	High fat diet (esp. saturated fat)	Linked to higher mortality and worse prognosis (RR = 1.3).
	Smoking	Controversial; increased risk, especially if smoking starts early; higher risk if combined with alcohol (RR = 1.54).

Table 3.
Risk factors for breast cancer [1].

DOI: http://dx.doi.org/10.5772/intechopen.1011885

Gene	Location	Gene type	Function/role	Pathogenic mechanism	Clinical implication
BRCA1	17q21	Tumor suppressor	DNA repair, cell cycle checkpoint	Mutation → genomic instability, apoptosis	↑ Risk of hereditary breast cancer (esp. triple-negative subtype)
BRCA2	13q12	Tumor suppressor	Homologous recombination via RAD51	Mutation → defective DNA repair	↑ Risk of hereditary breast cancer (luminal type, high-grade)
HER2 (ERBB2)	17q12	Oncogene	Tyrosine kinase receptor → proliferation	Amplification/overexpression	Found in ~20% of BC patients; poor prognosis; therapeutic target (trastuzumab)
EGFR (HER1)	7p12	Oncogene	Tyrosine kinase receptor → PI3K, MAPK, JNK signaling	Overexpression in TNBC & IBC	Associated with poor prognosis; potential target in TNBC
c-Myc	8q24	Oncogene	Transcription factor → regulates 15% of genome	Overexpression → uncontrolled proliferation	Associated with high-grade, invasive BC
Ras (H-, K-, N-ras)	H: 11p15K: 12p12N: 1p22	Oncogene	Small GTPase → signaling cascade activation	Missense mutations (rare in BC) or pathway hyperactivation	Involved in advanced disease and poor prognosis
BMI1	10p11.23	Oncogene	Regulates stem cell self-renewal	Synergizes with H-ras to promote invasion	Associated with tumor aggressiveness
RAD51/ DMC1	15q15.1/22q13.1	DNA repair genes	Homologous recombination (BRCA2 co-factors)	Deficient activity if BRCA2 is mutated	Impaired DNA repair contributes to carcinogenesis

Table 4.
Genes related to breast cancer [1].

3. Screening and diagnosis

Most countries have developed national breast cancer screening programs, due to the significant impact of breast cancer. Breast screening and diagnostic evaluations are different. Breast screening is conducted in asymptomatic women to identify potentially concerning abnormalities, though histopathological examination remains necessary for definitive breast cancer diagnosis. The screening approach is individualized based on each patient's specific risk factors and typically encompasses physical examination, risk evaluation, and imaging studies. The most commonly used imaging modality is mammography, although MRI is reserved for select high-risk cases [12].

The stage and the type of breast cancer play a crucial role in prognostic and treatment plan. In the U.S., out of the 250,000 breast cancer cases diagnosed annually, approximately 41,000 patients die from the disease. Therefore, the majority of patients do not die from breast cancer [13]. Geographic location significantly influences the 5-year relative survival rates for breast cancer. In developed regions like Japan and North America, survival rates are over 80%, but in less developed countries from Africa, this proportion falls below 40%. These proportions are largely influenced by the availability of financial support for both treatment and prevention, such as access to mammography screening [1].

4. Treatment strategies and breast reconstruction

Breast cancer treatment requires a multidisciplinary approach, involving collaboration among various specialists to achieve the best possible outcomes for the patient. The treatment of breast cancer has evolved over the years, both medically and surgically, leading to an important decrease in mortality. The goals of surgical treatment are to achieve local disease control, prevent locoregional recurrence, and improve overall survival. Almost 90% of patients with breast cancer diagnosis have early-stage disease and are eligible for surgical treatment. Surgical treatment of the breast can be divided into breast-conserving surgery and mastectomy, followed by oncoplastic reconstruction or breast reconstruction. In the last years, mastectomy rates, both unilateral and bilateral, have increased, even among women without genetic mutations. This trend is caused by the desire to achieve the most aesthetic result, reduce the risk for future cancer, and the expectation of improved quality of life [14].

As breast cancer rates continue to rise, concerns regarding postoperative aesthetics have become increasingly relevant to patients and clinicians alike. To improve patients' quality of life and enhance their self-image, advanced surgical techniques have been developed within oncological treatment, allowing for the integration of breast reconstruction procedures after mastectomy or oncoplastic surgery in cases of breast-conserving surgery. These surgical techniques do not compromise oncological safety; as a result, they have become an essential component of cancer care. However, about 10 years ago, only 33% of eligible women in the U.S. have chosen immediate breast reconstruction after mastectomy. This discrepancy highlighted a significant gap in access to care, patient education, and surgical evolution and availability [15].

In 2023, the American Society of Plastic Surgeons reported 117.512 immediate breast reconstructions and only 40,228 delayed breast reconstructions, representing 74.5% for immediate breast reconstruction. This significant evolution stems from enhanced surgical techniques and outcomes, advancement in mastectomy procedures, and improved patient education [16]. This pattern reflects the rising significance and expanding need for breast reconstruction procedures.

Breast reconstruction involves two phases: reconstruction of the breast mound and reconstruction of the nipple-areolar complex. Breast mound reconstruction can be achieved through implant-based methods or using autologous tissue from the patient's own body. The gold standard method for breast reconstruction, as considered by many plastic surgeons, is free DIEP (deep inferior epigastric perforator) flap breast reconstruction. One of the main advantages is high long-term satisfaction rates for patients and lower revision rates, especially in patients who previously had radiotherapy on the chest [16]. In 1979, Robbins performed the first breast reconstruction using a pedicled abdominal vertical flap, and in 1982, Hartrampf et al. adapted the technique with a horizontally oriented flap. Abdominal flap can be used to recreate the shape of the breast, utilizing the skin and adipose tissue of the lower abdomen. Flap elevation may be performed using two main techniques: one that spares the rectus abdominis muscle (DIEP free flap), and another that involves its inclusion (TRAM free flap). DIEP free flap has the advantage to preserve the muscle and the nerves, with lower morbidity on the abdominal wall [17]. The timing of breast reconstruction falls into two categories: immediate reconstruction, conducted simultaneously with the mastectomy procedure, and delayed reconstruction, performed in a subsequent operation after the mastectomy. Studies reported that immediate breast reconstruction has more advantages: reducing the number of surgical procedures, reducing recovery time, lower psychological impact, with better quality of life, and lower costs.

To achieve better aesthetic results with similar oncological control, surgical approach progresses to breast-conserving therapy with oncoplastic reconstruction and mastectomy with breast reconstruction. As a result, advancements in surgical practice have led to the development of skin-sparing and nipple-sparing mastectomy techniques. These approaches allow to preserve skin envelope, inframammary fold, and, in case of nipple-sparing mastectomy, nipple areola complex. The main concern for these techniques is the oncological control. The National Comprehensive Cancer Network recommends that nipple-sparing mastectomy can be done in patients with a distance between tumor and areola greater than 2 cm without nipple invasion [18].

A significant gap was demonstrated in education of the patients with breast cancer regarding breast reconstruction, which was highlighted in a recent survey conducted by The Harris Poll commissioned by the American Society of Plastic Surgeons (ASPS), which found that more than 50% of respondents reported limited knowledge of their reconstructive options [4, 11]. Furthermore, 62% of respondents did not know that it may be possible to regain sensation in the breast over time, and 73% of women were not informed that surgical costs are covered by insurance [19].

Surgical management of breast cancer has undergone significant evolution over time. The Halsted radical mastectomy, originally developed in the late nineteenth century, has been increasingly superseded by more tissue-sparing techniques. The current standard, the Madden modified radical mastectomy, involves removal of the breast tissue along with axillary lymph node dissection while preserving both the pectoralis major and minor muscles. Breast cancer surgery has evolved significantly over the past century. In 1972, John Madden introduced the modified radical mastectomy that preserved both pectoral muscles—marking a major shift from the more aggressive Halsted procedure used since 1894. Earlier attempts to expand the surgery, known as supraradical mastectomies, led to high complication rates without added benefit. As understanding of cancer biology and treatment improved, more conservative approaches became viable, offering similar oncologic safety with far better cosmetic outcomes. The adoption of the sentinel lymph node biopsy helped minimize unnecessary axillary dissections, significantly reducing complications such as lymphedema, numbness, and limited shoulder mobility. At the same time, oncoplastic surgery, which merges cancer removal with reconstructive techniques, enabled patients to benefit from procedures like nipple-sparing and skin-sparing mastectomies, improving both form and function [20].

The most prevalent form of this procedure today is simple mastectomy, which involves removal of the entire breast tissue along with the overlying skin and nipple-areolar complex. Some versions of this surgery aim to preserve as much skin as possible, to help with reconstruction performed later. In a skin-sparing mastectomy, most of the skin is kept intact. In a nipple-sparing mastectomy, the nipple and surrounding area are preserved. The radical mastectomy, in the past considered the gold standard in breast cancer surgery, involves en bloc resection of the entire breast tissue, associated axillary lymph nodes, and the underlying pectoral muscles. Due to its high morbidity and the development of less invasive (but equally effective) alternatives, this approach is now largely of historical interest and is not currently indicated in modern oncologic practice. Contemporary management of breast cancer has significantly evolved with the advancement of systemic therapies, including chemotherapy, targeted agents, and radiation therapy. Additionally, a more refined understanding of the biology and systemic nature of breast cancer has led to the widespread adoption of breast-conserving surgery (e.g., lumpectomy or partial mastectomy), where only the tumor combined with surrounding healthy tissue is excised. Nonetheless, mastectomy continues to play a central role in specific clinical scenarios, particularly when breast-conserving approaches are contraindicated or unfeasible. These indications may include multicentric disease, contraindications to radiation therapy, extensive ductal carcinoma in situ (DCIS), preference of the patient, or certain benign pathologies with high recurrence potential [21].

Robotic nipple-sparing mastectomy (R-NSM) has raised a growing interest in recent years. However, several critical questions remain unanswered: most notably, its oncological safety. Existing studies are limited by small patient cohorts and short follow-up periods, making it difficult to draw definitive conclusions about long-term cancer outcomes. These concerns are not unfounded, especially given the pre-existent experiences with minimally invasive radical hysterectomy [22]. That technique, initially adopted based on retrospective data, was later found to be inferior to open surgery in a randomized phase III trial that demonstrated significantly better survival outcomes in the open surgery group [23].

Beyond its oncological safety, there are several other key considerations when it comes to robotic nipple-sparing mastectomy (R-NSM), particularly the learning curve and cost-effectiveness of the procedure. Generally, surgeons tend to become more efficient with robotic techniques over time, as operative times shorten and the need to switch to open surgery decreases. However, this learning process can vary widely between individuals. One major factor is the surgeon's prior experience with minimally invasive surgery, something that many breast surgeons may not have. Formal training programs (often used in gastrointestinal surgery) can help, especially when they include tools like virtual reality simulations, hands-on practice with biotissue models, access to recorded procedures, and structured feedback. Thus, even these programs typically do not offer ways to measure how thoroughly breast tissue is removed, which is essential for ensuring the oncological effectiveness of the surgery [22].

Cost is another important issue. Robotic procedures come with a high price tag, because of several factors including the initial investment in the robotic platform, ongoing maintenance, single-use instruments, and often longer operating times. In more complex surgeries, where robotic techniques may reduce complications or lead to quicker recovery, these extra costs might be balanced out by better outcomes. However, that balance is harder to achieve with nipple-sparing mastectomies. These procedures involve minimal complications, and most patients can be discharged in 24 hours. Given this, the added expense of using a robot may not translate into significant medical or financial benefits [22].

Silicone gel breast implants were used for the first time for reconstruction in 1963 by Cronin and Gerow for a delayed breast reconstruction after a mastectomy, and in the 1970s, they also reported an immediate breast reconstruction with implants. First initiative to perform a prepectoral breast reconstruction was in the 1980s, but it was no longer pursued on account of high complication rates and poor aesthetic results and a total submuscular placement was preferred for breast reconstructions. The subpectoral placement, situated below the pectoralis major and serratus anterior muscles, exhibited considerable drawbacks. As a result, this technique progresses into the dual-plane approach, with implant position beneath the pectoralis major muscle in the upper pole and under the skin flap of acellular dermal matrix (ADM) in the lower pole [24].

Since its first use in 2001, Acellular dermal matrix has become an important component in breast surgery for correction of symmastia, rippling, and soft tissue deficits. Furthermore, ADMs are also used in implant-based immediate breast reconstruction with implant or tissue expander, for limiting the muscle dissection to create a dual-plane and lower rates of capsule contraction. Acellular dermal matrices are soft tissue grafts derived from human or animal skin, composed predominant of collagen and extracellular matrix components, by decellularization of tissue. An optimal ADM is not recognized as a foreign material by the human body and induces minimal inflammatory response, but should be revascularized and integrated by cells in the tissue. Even though it has notable advantages, including better control and definition in breast reconstruction, this technique also has limitations. These include higher risk of complications, like seroma formation, infection, or skin necrosis, and increased operative costs [25].

5. BIA-ALCL

In the recent years, the use of breast implants has increased in popularity, not only for aesthetic procedures, but also in reconstructive surgery. Although a few common complications may occur (such as seroma, hematoma, infection, or implant rupture) and are well documented, one rare but serious event has raised awareness: breast implant-associated anaplastic large cell lymphoma (BIA-ALCL). It is a CD30-positive T-cell lymphoma that typically arises in the fibrous capsule that surrounds the implant, especially associated with textured implants (with over 70% of reported cases related to this type of surface). The precise etiology still remains unclear, even though it is believed to be multifactorial, involving host immune responses and implant characteristics [26]. Despite its low global incidence (which cannot be exactly set, but it is estimated to vary between 1 in 3817 and 1 in 30,000), the condition has drawn increased attention from international health authorities, particularly after data revealed a disproportionate number of cases associated with Allergan implants. As of mid-2024, the FDA had recorded 1380 reports of BIA-ALCL for medical devices, including 64 deaths and underscoring the need for vigilance despite the rarity of the disease [26–28]. The clinical presentation of this disease is variable, with the majority of patients presenting with late-onset seroma or even capsular masses that occur approximately 8–10 years after implantation. Complete surgical excision represents the main strategy of treatment, with favorable outcomes reported in most cases. However, a few drawbacks such as limitations in post-marketing surveillance data, inconsistencies regarding implant texture classification, and insufficient long-term studies on this subject (particularly on newer implant types such as polyurethane implants), obstruct the formation of universal guidelines. Consequently, current recommendations emphasize individualized patient management, thorough informed consent, and ongoing monitoring, rather than routine explantation in asymptomatic individuals (**Table 5**) [26].

In the United Kingdom, four of ten women with breast cancer go through mastectomy owing to individual preference or oncological indication. In response to this growing burden, breast reconstruction has gained an essential role in breast cancer care. The first breast reconstruction following a mastectomy was performed in 1895,

Category	Key information
Definition	Rare T-cell lymphoma ($CD30^{+}$), which arises in the capsule surrounding breast implants.
Etiology	Multifactorial; not fully understood.
Incidence	Ranges from 1 in 3817 to 1 in 30,000.
Total reported cases (worldwide)	1619 cases reported by ASPS; 1380 MDRs reported to FDA globally (as of April 17, 2025).
Total reported cases in the U.S.	456 confirmed or suspected cases (as of April 17, 2025).
Median age at diagnosis	53 years.
Latency period	Typically 8–9 years post-implantation.
Clinical Presentation	Pain, asymmetry, seroma, capsular mass, rash, lymphadenopathy.
Most common cause of death	Capsular masses (39%).
Survival/Prognosis	93% disease-free survival at 3 years post-treatment.
Treatment	Complete capsulectomy and implant removal.
Implant surface association	73% of BIA-ALCL cases involve textured implants; only 3% smooth implants (often with unclear history).
Implant fill type	67% silicone-filled; 26% saline-filled.
Implant indication	Equal distribution of cosmetic (16%) and reconstructive (16%) purposes; 68% unspecified.
Most implicated manufacturer	Allergan (86% of cases); Mentor (5%), Sientra (2%), Others (1%), Unknown (6%).
Incidence rate - Allergan	1 in 2207.
Geographical distribution	43% U.S., 47% non-U.S., 10% unspecified.
FDA MDR system role	Key post-market surveillance tool, limited by under-reporting and incomplete data.
Polyurethane-coated implants	Limited data; suspected to have higher BIA-ALCL association, but evidence is inconclusive.

Table 5.
Summary of key findings on breast implant-associated anaplastic large cell lymphoma (BIA-ALCL) [26].

by transplanting a lipoma from the lumbar region to the chest [24]. According to the American Society of Plastic Surgeons (ASPS), the annual number of breast reconstructions performed has a significant upward trend, with a 48.3% rise from 106,338 procedures in 2015 to 157,740 in 2023, underscoring the growing demand for this type of surgery [29]. The majority of breast reconstructions, with over 80%, are performed using implants, making this the most widely adopted method. Its main advantages include a shorter operative time, faster recovery, and the absence of donor site morbidity. The evolution of breast reconstruction techniques has followed irregular path. Initially, the prepectoral implant technique was used; however, due to a higher risk of complications, the approach shifted toward submuscular implant placement [30]. Recently, the prepectoral approach has regained popularity and become the main performed technique for breast reconstruction, with 106,380 prepectoral breast reconstructions completed in the U.S. in 2023. Approximately two-thirds (67%) of reconstructions were prepectoral, while submuscular reconstructions represented the remaining 33% [29]. The technique spares the pectoral muscle from dissection and avoids animation deformity, pain, and shoulder dysfunction. Improvements in conservative mastectomy, particularly the preservation of subcutaneous tissue in the mastectomy flap, play a crucial role in minimizing the complications associated with the initial applications of prepectoral breast reconstruction [31].

Polyurethane implants offer remarkable aesthetic outcomes with no major complications and are cost-effective because they do not require the use of acellular dermal matrix. These types of implants have "Velcro Effect," the ability for adhesion and attach firmly to the breast prepectoral pocket: superficial fascia of pectoralis major and mastectomy flap. This capacity to adhere to surrounding tissue provides stability for the implant and lowers the risk of seroma. In addition, the stable position of the implants offers lower rates of revision surgery and leads to long-lasting and consistent results [31].

6. Technique prepectoral breast reconstruction

Among the many techniques described for prepectoral implant-based reconstruction, the author adopted the following procedure. After the mastectomy is performed, meticulous hemostasis is achieved. The mastectomy flaps are then evaluated, and in most cases, we assess their vascularity using indocyanine green (ICG) fluorescence imaging.

If the flaps are well vascularized, we proceed with prepectoral reconstruction using a polyurethane-coated implant. In the author's opinion, polyurethane implants are the optimal choice for this type of reconstruction due to their "Velcro effect," which provides excellent implant stability. This approach eliminates the need for acellular dermal matrix (ADM), thereby reducing the risk of ADM-related complications and lowering overall surgical costs.

The author considers that the benefits of ADM are limited in this context. He also believes that microtextured implants are not suitable for placement in the prepectoral pocket, as they are prone to shifting, making it difficult to predict long-term outcomes.

Once the implant is carefully positioned in the prepectoral space, a surgical drain is placed, and the implant's position is re-checked. It is crucial to ensure that the polyurethane implant is placed in an optimal position from the outset, as it will not migrate over time. The implant should be positioned as low as possible to avoid visible contour irregularities and achieve the best aesthetic outcome.

In the second scenario, if areas of the mastectomy skin flap demonstrate inadequate perfusion, those regions are surgically excised. Breast reconstruction is then performed using a tissue expander placed in a subpectoral pocket, typically under the pectoralis major muscle, and, in some cases, extended with coverage from the serratus anterior fascia at the lower pole.

This technique offers the advantage of reduced pressure on the mastectomy flaps, thereby decreasing the risk of skin necrosis or wound dehiscence—complications that could otherwise result in implant exposure and necessitate implant removal. After the prosthesis is placed, a surgical drain is positioned within the pocket. Subcutaneous sutures are performed using 2/0 and 3/0 Dacron, followed by intradermal sutures with 3/0 Monocryl. The incision is then covered with Omnistrips and a sterile dressing.

With the growing interest in and integration of breast reconstruction as part of breast cancer treatment, aesthetic outcomes have become a major focus. Advances in surgical techniques now make it possible to reconstruct a breast that closely resembles the natural one. Lipofilling has emerged as an innovative technique that significantly enhances the aesthetic result by correcting contour irregularities, filling tissue defects, and improving rippling through the thickening of mastectomy flaps. The main concern for this technique was the oncological safety, which was studied in the last 20 years, and these concerns are not supported by high-quality evidence. Lipofilling is a surgical technique that replaces the autologous fat, usually harvested from areas with excess volume, such as the abdomen, thighs, and even the medial part of the knees in thin patients, and injected in areas requiring volumization. At the level of the reconstructed breast, the autogenous fat offers multiple advantages: avoiding the risk of allergic reaction and rejection by using autogenous tissue, improving the texture and the aspects of the breast, enhancing contour and symmetry. This procedure can be performed in multiple sessions and allows for a noticeable increase in volume and projection. Additionally, patients benefit the reshaping of donor site areas, like abdomen or thighs with minimal scars and easy recovery [32].

Transferred fat is an active tissue composed of different structures: adipocytes, fibroblasts, endothelial cells, and adipogenic progenitor cells. Adipose-derived stem cells (ASCs) give functional advantage to this technique for regeneration. ASCs are multipotent mesenchymal stem cells and are present in the stromal vascular fraction (SVF) of adipose tissue. These structures play a crucial role in regenerative medicine, being able to restore the subcutaneous tissue and dermis. Thanks to their capacity for neocollagenesis and neoangiogenesis, these cells enhance dermal thickening, resulting in improved skin quality. This approach has proven to be an effective therapeutic option, especially in patients who experienced late adverse effects of oncologic radiation therapy [33].

There are several indications for fat grafting in breast surgery. It is indicated to correct soft tissue defects, also to achieve a better aesthetic, and scar correction. It can be applied after breast conservative surgery, in implant-based reconstruction, and in some cases for entire breast reconstruction with multiple sessions of lipofilling.

The main concern for this procedure is the oncological safety, due to the ASCs, biologically active cellular progenitors, which can increase the risk of recurrence. Endothelial progenitor cells are found in human white adipose tissue (WAT), which is a very rich source of CD45-CD34+ EPCs. These cells have the ability to differentiate into endothelial cells that can produce endothelial tubes and enhanced tumor vascularization that can lead to stimulating tumor progression at both the primary and metastatic levels [34]. Research conducted by Martin-Padura et al. [34] demonstrates that co-injection of adipose-derived mesenchymal stem cells (ADSCs) with tumor cells in murine models led to accelerated tumor growth. This effect appears to be mediated by the secretion of growth and angiogenic factors, which promote tumor cell proliferation [34]. However, other studies have denied this conclusion. Studies conducted by Goto et al., Gebremeskel et al., Tsuji et al., and Silva et al. reported that mice receiving fat grafts revealed reduced tumor volumes, suggesting a potential protective effect against tumor growth [35]. A systematic review by Rodrigo Gonçalves et al. evaluated 15 observational studies to investigate the oncological safety of autologous fat grafting (AFG) in breast cancer patients. The findings indicated no significant differences in overall survival (OS), disease-free survival (DFS), or local recurrence rates between patients who underwent AFG as part of breast reconstruction and those who did not. The review included over 2331 participants [35]. Despite most studies demonstrating oncological safety, Cell-assisted lipotransfer (CAL) must be performed with prudence, due to concerns related to oncological safety. This technique is used to enhance the effectiveness of autologous fat grafting by improving graft survival and retention. This also led to reducing common adverse effects such as fibrosis, pseudocyst formation, and calcification [33].

Autologous fat graft also may lead to complications such as: calcifications, fat necrosis, and cyst formation, due to suboptimal incorporation of fat graft. The viability of fat graft and integration within the host tissue is critical for a positive outcome. The formation of necrotic cysts and calcification may complicate oncological surveillance, as they can appear radiologically similar to recurrent disease on mammography and PET-CT imaging. To avoid this complication and enhance the integration of fat grafting, surgeons perform small volume on lipofilling, in multiple sessions. Additionally, fat graft injection is performed with a blunt cannula, however when its insertion can damage the underlying breast implant [3].

7. Lipofilling technique used by the author

Various approaches can be employed when performing lipofilling in breast reconstruction. Some surgeons opt for primary lipofilling, conducted during the same surgical session as the mastectomy, or as part of secondary reconstruction, prior to the placement of a tissue expander.

The author prefers to perform lipofilling as a secondary procedure, thereby avoiding additional trauma to the flaps, which may already be compromised in terms of vascularity. Although performing lipofilling before expander-based reconstruction may offer benefits for tissue regeneration, in cases where the tissues are significantly damaged—especially due to radiotherapy—the author generally chooses autologous tissue reconstruction, which provides the added advantage of excising irradiated tissue and replacing it with healthy, well-vascularized tissue.

Typically, lipofilling is carried out 3–6 months after implant-based reconstruction. The procedure is performed under general anesthesia, allowing for improved patient comfort and optimal fat harvesting conditions.

Initially, 500 ml of Klein's solution (1 ml adrenaline 1 mg/ml in 1000 ml normal saline) is infiltrated into the donor area. After a waiting period of 7–20 minutes, fat is harvested using a Tonnard Harvester cannula.

Following purification, the fat is injected with precision, using a superficial placement technique to avoid any risk of damaging the breast implant. To optimize graft survival and reduce resorption, fat is injected at a ratio of 1 ml per 10 linear centimeters. The injection is performed in small, evenly distributed aliquots to promote proper vascularization and integration of the graft. This technique helps to minimize complications such as oil cyst formation and fat necrosis (**Table 6**).

Category	Details	References
Patient Expectations	Growing demand for natural-feeling results post-reconstruction.	[3]
Role of Fat Grafting (FG)	FG improves implant rippling and overall aesthetic outcomes when added to IBR.	[3, 4]
Medical Benefits of FG	Helps in cases with capsular contracture, wound healing, and mitigates radiation-induced fibrosis.	[3, 5]
Complication Rate	Fat grafting has a lower rate of surgical complications compared to other methods.	[3]
Satisfaction Rate	High satisfaction among both patients and surgeons.	[3]
Oncological Safety Concerns	Initially debated due to fears of oncogenic potential and confusion with neoplastic calcifications on imaging.	[4]
Current Evidence	Studies have disproven concerns; FG is currently a widely accepted adjunct to IBR.	[6]

Table 6.
Overview of fat grafting in implant-based breast reconstruction.

Breast reconstruction gained a significant role in breast cancer treatment. The technique that combines polyurethane-coated prepectoral implant breast reconstruction with sequential lipofilling represents an innovative, safe, and effective strategy that enhances the advantages of both implant-based and autologous techniques.

Prepectoral placement of implants preserves the muscle integrity and avoids the animation deformities. Polyurethane surface with Velcro effect offers stability and enhances integration of the implant. Sequential lipofilling offers a significant improvement in achieving both aesthetic and functional outcomes in patients with prepectoral implant breast reconstruction. This surgical approach became a standard practice in modern breast reconstruction with high levels of patient satisfaction and long-term reconstructive success.

Author details

Ioan-Constantin Pop[1,2]*, Maximilian-Vlad Muntean[1,2] and Radu-Alexandru Ilies[3]

1 Department of Plastic Surgery, "Prof. Dr. I. Chiricuță" Institute of Oncology, Cluj-Napoca, Romania

2 Department of Plastic and Reconstructive Surgery, "Iuliu Hațieganu" University of Medicine and Pharmacy, Cluj-Napoca, Romania

3 Faculty of Medicine, "Iuliu Hațieganu" University of Medicine and Pharmacy, Cluj-Napoca, Romania

*Address all correspondence to: drp.ionut@gmail.com

References

[1] Sun YS, Zhao Z, Yang ZN, Xu F, Lu HJ, Zhu ZY, et al. Risk factors and preventions of breast cancer. International Journal of Biological Sciences. 2017;**13**(11):1387-1397. DOI: 10.7150/ijbs.21635

[2] Key TJ, Verkasalo PK, Banks E. Epidemiology of breast cancer. The Lancet Oncology. 2001;**2**(3):133-140. DOI: 10.1016/S1470-2045(00)00254-0

[3] Allen, Gabriel MYN. Spear's Surgery of the Breast: Principles and Art. 4th ed. Philadelphia, PA: Lippincott Williams & Wilkins (Wolters Kluwer Health); 2020

[4] Turner A, Abu-Ghname A, Davis MJ, Winocour SJ, Hanson SE, Chu CK. Fat grafting in breast reconstruction. Seminars in Plastic Surgery. 2020;**34**(1):17-23

[5] Calabrese S, Zingaretti N, De Francesco F, Riccio M, De Biasio F, Massarut S, et al. Long-term impact of lipofilling in hybrid breast reconstruction: Retrospective analysis of two cohorts. European Journal of Plastic Surgery. 2020;**43**:257-268

[6] Delay E, Garson S, Tousson G, Sinna R. Fat injection to the breast: Technique, results, and indications based on 880 procedures over 10 years. Aesthetic Surgery Journal. 2009;**29**(5):360-376

[7] Waks AG, Winer EP. Breast cancer treatment: A review. Journal of the American Medical Association. 2019;**321**(3):288-300. DOI: 10.1001/jama.2018.19323

[8] Britt KL, Cuzick J, Phillips KA. Key steps for effective breast cancer prevention. Nature Reviews Cancer. 2020;**20**(8):417-436. DOI: 10.1038/s41568-020-0266-x. Epub 2020 Jun 11

[9] Kamińska M, Ciszewski T, Łopacka-Szatan K, Miotła P, Starosławska E. Breast cancer risk factors. Menopause Review/Przegląd Menopauzalny. 2015;**14**(3):196-202. DOI: 10.5114/pm.2015.54346. Epub 2015 Sep 30

[10] Sauter ER. Breast cancer prevention: Current approaches and future directions. European Journal of Breast Health. 2018;**14**(2):64-71. DOI: 10.5152/ejbh.2018.3978

[11] Nathanson KL, Wooster R, Weber BL. Breast cancer genetics: What we know and what we need. Nature Medicine. 2001;**7**(5):552-556. DOI: 10.1038/87876. Erratum in: Nat Med 2001;7(6):749. Nathanson KN [corrected to Nathanson KL]

[12] Huzarski T, Górecka-Szyld B, Huzarska J, Psut-Muszyńska G, Wilk G, Sibilski R, et al. Screening with magnetic resonance imaging, mammography and ultrasound in women at average and intermediate risk of breast cancer. Hereditary Cancer in Clinical Practice. 2017;**15**:4. DOI: 10.1186/s13053-017-0064-y

[13] Waks AG, Winer EP. Breast cancer treatment. Journal of the American Medical Association. 2019;**321**(3):316. DOI: 10.1001/jama.2018.20751

[14] Lovelace DL, McDaniel LR, Golden D. Long-term effects of breast cancer surgery, treatment, and survivor care. Journal of Midwifery & Women's Health. 2019;**64**(6):713-724. DOI: 10.1111/jmwh.13012. Epub 2019 Jul 19

[15] American Society of Plastic Surgeons. Plastic Surgery Statistics

Report 2023. Arlington (VA): American Society of Plastic Surgeons; 2023. Available from: https://www.plasticsurgery.org/documents/news/statistics/2023/plastic-surgery-statistics-report-2023.pdfen.wikipedia.org+2

[16] Opsomer D, Vyncke T, Depypere B, Stillaert F, Blondeel P, Van Landuyt K. Lumbar flap versus the gold standard: Comparison to the DIEP flap. Plastic and Reconstructive Surgery. 2020;**145**(4):706e-714e. DOI: 10.1097/PRS.0000000000006681

[17] Tomita K, Kubo T. Recent advances in surgical techniques for breast reconstruction. International Journal of Clinical Oncology. 2023;**28**:841-846. DOI: 10.1007/s10147-023-02313-1

[18] Clarijs ME, Peeters NJMCV, van Dongen SAF, Koppert LB, Pusic AL, Mureau MAM, et al. Quality of life and complications after nipple- versus skin-sparing mastectomy followed by immediate breast reconstruction: A systematic review and meta-analysis. Plastic and Reconstructive Surgery. 2023;**152**(1):12e-24e. DOI: 10.1097/PRS.0000000000010155. Epub 2023 Jun 29

[19] American Society of Plastic Surgeons. Survey: Many U.S. Women Lack Basic Information on Life After Mastectomy. 2022. Available from: https://www.plasticsurgery.org/news/press-releases/survey-many-us-women-lack-basic-information-on-life-after-mastectomy

[20] Plesca M, Bordea C, El Houcheimi B, Ichim E, Blidaru A. Evolution of radical mastectomy for breast cancer. Journal of Medicine and Life. 2016;**9**(2):183-186

[21] Goethals A, Menon G, Rose J. Mastectomy. In: StatPearls. Treasure Island (FL): StatPearls Publishing; 2025 [Accessed: 10 November 2024]

[22] Morrow M. Robotic mastectomy: The next major advance in breast cancer surgery? The British Journal of Surgery. 2021;**108**(3):233-234. DOI: 10.1093/bjs/znab010

[23] Ramirez PT, Frumovitz M, Pareja R, Lopez A, Vieira M, Ribeiro R, et al. Minimally invasive versus abdominal radical hysterectomy for cervical cancer. The New England Journal of Medicine. 2018;**379**:1895-1904

[24] Chopra S, Al-Ishaq Z, Vidya R. The journey of prepectoral breast reconstruction through time. World Journal of Plastic Surgery. 2021;**10**(2):3-13. DOI: 10.29252/wjps.10.2.3

[25] Hallberg H, Rafnsdottir S, Selvaggi G, Strandell A, Samuelsson O, Stadig I, et al. Benefits and risks with acellular dermal matrix (ADM) and mesh support in immediate breast reconstruction: A systematic review and meta-analysis. Journal of Plastic Surgery and Hand Surgery. 2018;**52**(3):130-147. DOI: 10.1080/2000656X.2017.1419141

[26] Muntean M, Ilies RA, Pop IC, Urian L, Vlad IC, Achimas-Cadariu P. Unveiling the controversy: A literature review on the link between textured implants and breast implant-associated anaplastic large cell lymphoma (BIA-ALCL). Journal of Clinical Medicine. 2025;**14**:3902. DOI: 10.3390/jcm14113902

[27] BIA-ALCL Resources. 2020. Available from: https://www.plasticsurgery.org/for-medical-professionals/health-policy/bia-alcl-physician-resources/by-the-numbers [Accessed: 13 May 2025]

[28] Medical Device Reports of Breast Implant-Associated Anaplastic Large Cell Lymphoma. 2025. Available from: https://www.fda.gov/medical-devices/breast-implants/

medical-device-reports-breast-implant-associated-anaplastic-large-cell-lymphoma [Accessed: 13 May 2025]

[29] American Society of Plastic Surgeons. Reconstructive Breast Procedures (with Age Distribution) 2023. Arlington (VA): American Society of Plastic Surgeons; 2023. Available from: https://www.plasticsurgery.org/documents/news/statistics/2023/reconstructive-breast-procedures-age-2023.pdf

[30] Hong SE, Kang D. Navigating the pandemic: Shifts in breast reconstruction trends and surgical decision-making in the United States. Journal of Clinical Medicine. 2024;**13**:4168. DOI: 10.3390/jcm13144168

[31] Salgarello M, Pagliara D, Barone Adesi L, Visconti G, Wild JB, Matey P. Direct to implant breast reconstruction with prepectoral micropolyurethane foam-coated implant: Analysis of patient satisfaction. Clinical Breast Cancer. 2021;**21**(4):e454-e461. DOI: 10.1016/j.clbc.2021.01.015. Epub 2021 Jan 23

[32] Kasem A, Wazir U, Headon H, Mokbel K. Breast lipofilling: A review of current practice. Archives of Plastic Surgery. 2015;**42**(2):126-130. DOI: 10.5999/aps.2015.42.2.126. Epub 2015 Mar 16

[33] Simonacci F, Bertozzi N, Grieco MP, Grignaffini E, Raposio E. Autologous fat transplantation for breast reconstruction: A literature review. Annals of Medicine and Surgery (London). 2016;**12**:94-100. DOI: 10.1016/j.amsu.2016.11.012

[34] Martin-Padura I, Gregato G, Marighetti P, Mancuso P, Calleri A, Corsini C, et al. The white adipose tissue used in lipotransfer procedures is a rich reservoir of $CD34^+$ progenitors able to promote cancer progression. Cancer Research. 2012;**72**(1):325-334. DOI: 10.1158/0008-5472.CAN-11-1739. Epub 2011 Nov 3

[35] Goncalves R, Mota BS, Sobreira-Lima B, et al. The oncological safety of autologous fat grafting: A systematic review and meta-analysis. BMC Cancer. 2022;**22**:391. DOI: 10.1186/s12885-022-09485-5

Chapter 9

A Plastic Surgeon's Perspective on the Management of Complicated Cases of Hidradenitis Suppurativa

Shilpi Karmakar and Ramani Saradha

Abstract

Hidradenitis suppurativa is a chronic inflammatory and recurrent cutaneous disorder that involves the apocrine glands. Axilla and inguinal regions are rich in these glands. Wide excision that involves surgical margins beyond the clinical extent of disease is recommended in Hurley stages II and III, in order to completely eliminate the disease and to prevent recurrence. After excision, these areas must be reconstructed with flaps. The various flaps that are possible for axilla resurfacing are parascapular, lateral thoracic artery perforator, thoracodorsal artery perforator, medial arm, posterior arm, and flaps. The various flaps that are possible for resurfacing of inguinal and anogenital region are anterolateral thigh, tensor fascia lata, rectus femoris, rectus abdominis, gracilis, and medial thigh flaps. In recent times, dermal templates are gaining popularity because of their versatility and ease of use. The planning of these flaps, advantages, and limitations is highlighted in this chapter.

Keywords: hidradenitis, axilla, apocrine, contracture, fascia, hair

1. Introduction

Recurrent lesions affecting the infundibular terminal follicles are a hallmark of Hidradenitis Suppurativa (HS), a chronic inflammatory skin condition [1]. Inflammation and the development of nodules, sinuses, abscesses, and fistulae are linked to it. It affects the axillary, inguinal, and anogenital skin regions that contain apocrine glands [1]. The Hurley clinical staging system classifies patients with HS into three levels of disease severity [1].

Stage I—abscess formation with no sinus tracts/scarring.

Stage II—repeated abscess formation along with sinus tracts and scarring which presents as either a single or separate multiple lesions.

Stage III—involvement that is diffuse or nearly diffuse, with numerous linked sinus tracts and abscesses across the entire region.

The various therapeutic options include: antibiotics, surgical techniques, and biologic therapies. Recent research suggests that starting medical treatment early can improve outcomes and reduce scarring, highlighting a critical "window of

IntechOpen

opportunity" in HS treatment. In a patient who seeks treatment within the therapeutic window of opportunity, current guidelines favor early surgical intervention in addition to medical therapy [2]. This is because systemic therapy alone might not result in total remission of sinus tract inflammation. Medical therapy aids by preparing the wound for optimal healing and encouraging a more distinct division between damaged and healthy tissue during surgery [3]. In order to avoid persistent inflammation in the skin, which might result in the formation of new lesions, total remission must be achieved [4]. Thus, the optimal therapeutic standard is a combination of medical therapy and surgery. The window of opportunity concept applies to both medical treatment and surgery. Antibiotics help by reducing the surgical area, preventing recurrence, and stopping disease progression at an earlier stage, and early surgery of symptomatic inflammatory lesions reduces fibrosis and the morbidity due to scarring. The type of surgery and the surgical methods employed affect the recurrence rates.

The only biological therapy for HS that has FDA approval is adalimumab. This drug is the first line of treatment for patients with moderate-to-severe sickness of age 12 years and above. It is a human recombinant IgG1 monoclonal antibody that targets the pro-inflammatory cytokine TNF-alpha [5]. The commonly prescribed dosage is 40 mg weekly and can be used continuously if tolerated [6]. Patients are unlikely to benefit from further treatment if they do not improve after 12 weeks [7].

Other monoclonal antibiotics used in practice include:

Infliximab—Chimeric monoclonal TNF-alpha antibody.

Apremilast—Phosphodiesterase-4 inhibitor.

Anakinra—Il-1 receptor inhibitor.

Secukinumab—IL-17 inhibitor.

Ustekinumab.

Etanercept [8].

——————————.

Surgical treatment of HS includes deroofing of small abscess, incision and drainage of abscess, sinus tract, or a nodule, electrosurgical incision of sinus tract, and excision of lesions. For minor defects, primary closure by mobilizing the surrounding lax skin might be possible. For moderate to significant defects, either one of the methods of closure—skin graft, flap, or dermal template with skin graft—must be used.

The success of primary closure depends on the tension of the closure. The more mobilization needed for closure, the more devascularization of the skin happens. The balance necessary between the undermining required to close a defect and the tension on the suture line is a delicate one. Added to the tension of closure is the tension due to movements of adjacent joints. While closing a defect, joint positioning must be carefully considered. Neglect of these considerations contributes to the high rates of suture dehiscence, reported by Mandal et al. and Ovadja et al. [3, 8].

Skin grafting is a good option when the defect is far from joints. Placing skin grafts over joints or just adjacent to joints is a perilous venture. With good intraoperative practices, such as meticulous hemostasis, ensuring vascularity of the bed, quilting of graft, infection prevention, and strict postoperative protocols, consisting of initial immobilzation, followed by massage, splintage, and physiotherapy, skin grafting is an economical, time-saving, and easy option. However, it is easier said than done. In the hands of most authors, engraftment rate remains uncertain [9]. The disadvantages of poor color match, dry and inelastic texture, chances of poor graft take, and possibility of secondary contracture have significantly restricted the utility of skin grafts in this condition [10].

It is highly recommended to do a wide excision with surgical margins that extend outside the clinical boundaries of the disease in cases of resistant and severe Hurley stages II and III. This approach aims to eliminate the disease and prevent recurrence [11]. The entire hair-bearing skin up to the level of fascia should be excised [11]. The surgery should be done along with appropriate antibiotic administration, in line with the French Society of Dermatology guidelines [1].

Since the involved areas are adjacent to the joints, they must not be left unreconstructed [1]. Besides long healing time, requiring complex and costly dressings, repeated scar breakdown, the development of contractures, unstable scar, and Marjolin's ulcer are serious concerns [12]. Recurrence rates of hidradenitis in areas left for healing by secondary intention are as high as 11 to 37.5% [13, 14].

Flaps are the procedure of choice after excision of the affected tissue. By giving a good well-vascularized tissue cover, scars are placed outside the joint folds, and the range of motion of the adjoining joints is maintained. They shorten the healing time and duration of hospital stay. The complication rate is also reduced [15]. Flaps are increasingly being used to treat hidradenitis suppurativa, and every surgeon should be well-versed with some of the flaps used in these regions.

A flap is a segment of tissue that is transferred into a defect while maintaining its blood flow. Based on their blood supply, flaps are divided into two categories: random pattern flaps, which depend on the dermal and subcutaneous vascular plexus, and axial flaps, which are supplied by a named artery [15].

Based on the composition, flaps are classified as:

1. Cutaneous

2. Fasciocutaneous/adipofascial

3. Musculocutaneous/muscle

Based on the location of the source blood vessel, flaps are divided into:

1. Free flaps: tissue is raised at a distant site and reperfused through vascular anastomosis.

2. Regional flaps: nonadjacent tissue near the defect is moved into the wound, preserving the vascular pedicle.

3. Local flaps: adjacent tissue is used to cover the wound.

2. Local flaps

Local flaps can be termed to as advancement, rotation, or transposition flaps depending on the predominant primary movement needed for transfer.

2.1 Rotation flap

Rotation flaps are curvilinear-shaped pivotal flaps. They are positioned directly next to the defect [16]. The line that runs from the flap base to a distal point along the curvilinear border has the highest tension for wound closure (**Figure 1**).

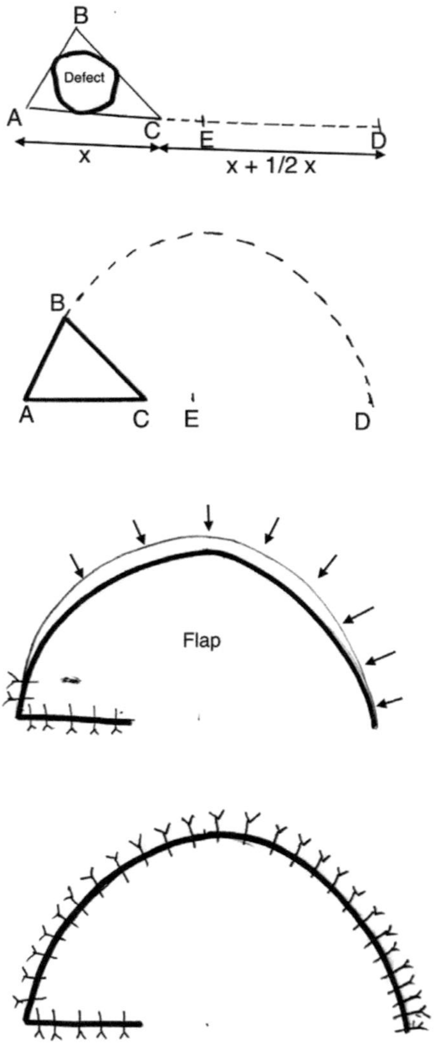

Figure 1.
Planning of rotation flap.

Triangle-shaped defects are ideal for rotation flaps. To achieve the best results with rotation flaps, defects can be adjusted into triangular forms through de-epithelialization or conservative excision of surrounding normal tissue [16]. When appropriately designed, the flap circumference is around four times the base of the triangle-shaped defect [16]. Thus, the flap has a broad-base and reliable vascularity. Its design and positioning offers great flexibility.

2.2 Transposition flap

Transposition flaps are linear in design as opposed to rotation flaps, which are curvilinear and the secondary defect of the flap donor site needs to be grafted [16]. Along a vector from the pivotal point to the furthest point on the flap border, the wound closure tension is maximum (**Figure 2**).

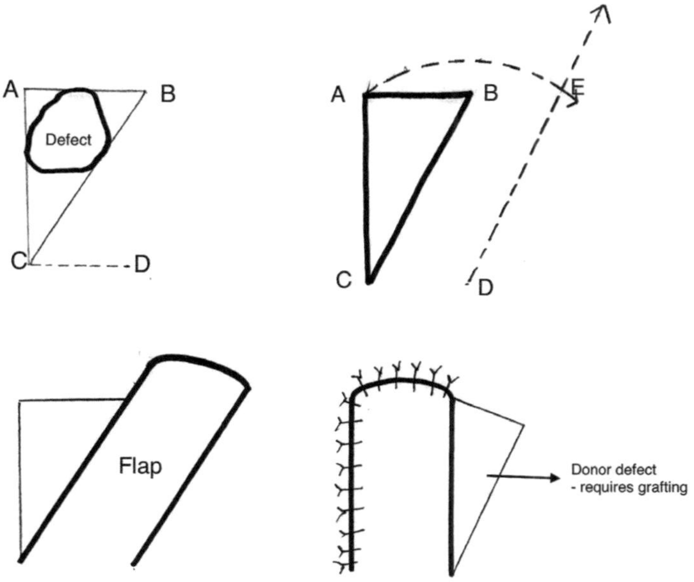

Figure 2.
Planning of transposition flap.

2.3 Advancement flap

Small- to medium-sized defects can be effectively repaired with the V-Y advancement flap. An advancement flap that is raised in the shape of a V and closed, giving a shape of Y, is called a V-Y advancement flap (**Figure 3**). The success of the V-Y flap

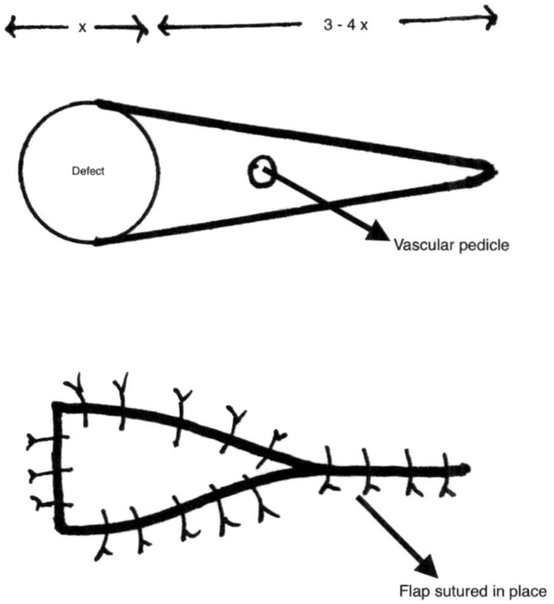

Figure 3.
V-Y advancement flap.

depends on the maintenance of a robust vascular pedicle. For hidradenitis suppurativa of the axilla, reconstruction can be performed using a V-Y fascioutaneous advancement flap from the lateral aspect of chest in case of smaller defects or a combination of 2 V-Y advancement flaps from the lateral chest and medial arm. Multiple direct cutaneous perforators from the pectoral branch of the acromio-thoracic artery, the lateral thoracic artery, and the thoracodorsal artery supply the lateral chest wall.

Five to six fasciocutaneous perforators supply give cutaneous supply to medial aspect of upper arm. These perforators originate from brachial artery and branches of brachial artery to the biceps, superior ulnar collateral artery, and, if present, the middle ulnar collateral artery. At the level of the deep fascia, the perforators spread out over triceps and biceps after emerging along the medial intermuscular septum. These flaps are thin and pliable and maintain the contour of the axilla [17].

3. Regional flaps

3.1 Axilla

While planning flap for reconstruction of axillary defects, the unique features of the axilla have to be kept in mind:

- A distinct concave shape that is difficult to replicate [18].
- In order to avoid a bulky reconstruction, the thickness of the flap should be suitable.
- Accuracy in the amount of skin is crucial to prevent excesses and retractions.
- Close relation to a joint, which has a wide range of movements.
- Placing scars such that they are as hidden as possible [18].

3.1.1 Parascapular flap

The parascapular flap is raised as a fasciocutaneous flap, overlying the lateral border of the scapula, from the posterolateral chest wall [19]. This can be raised as a flap due to wide caliber of the vessel, anatomic consistency, and the long length of vascular pedicle. It is based on the descending branch of the circumflex scapular branch of the subscapular artery. The emerging point of the vascular pedicle is marked by the omotricipital space. With finger palpation, this area—which is situated between the teres major below, the teres minor above, and the long head of the triceps laterally—feels like a depression [19].

The descending branch follows the lateral edge of the scapula as it descends toward its tip. The flap central axis is represented by the lateral edge of the scapula. The pedicle emergence and the flap superior margin are both marked at the same level. About 25–30 cm from the upper margin, the lower edge is delineated [19]. The donor defect can be closed if up to 8–10 cm wide. A skin graft is required to cover the donor location if the flap is wider (**Table 1** and **Figure 4**) [19].

Advantage	Disadvantages
The texture, color, and thinness of the flap skin are comparable to those of the axilla.	The flap is insensate.
The vascular source is constant, long and of wide caliber.	Flap harvest is possible only in prone or lateral position.
In most cases, there is no need for postoperative splints and the shoulder joint can be mobilized early.	It is generally non-hair bearing.
There is no functional morbidity.	

Table 1.
Advantages and disadvantages of Parascapular flap.

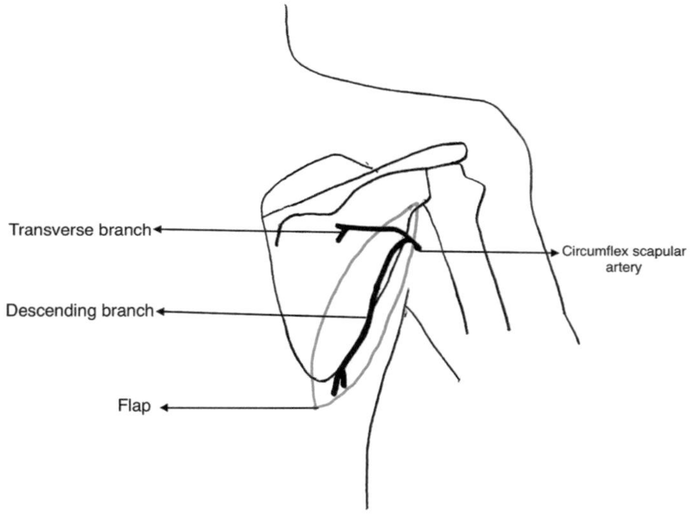

Figure 4.
Planning of parascapular flap.

3.1.2 Thoracodorsal artery perforator (TDAP) flap

Angrigiani et al. demonstrated the preservation of latissimus dorsi muscle while using a cutaneous flap fashioned from the thoracodorsal artery perforator branches [20]. The thoracodorsal artery and venae comitantes constitute the central vascular supply for latissimus dorsi muscle (**Figure 5**) [21]. The subscapular artery is its source vessel. The thoracodorsal vessels split into the descending branch and the horizontal branch after supplying the serratus muscle branch [14]. The descending branch follows an intramuscular course for 2–3 cm and gives 2 or 3 skin perforators. In the harvest of TDAP flap, the most proximal perforator enters the subcutaneous tissue at a place that is 2–3 cm behind the muscle lateral edge and 8 cm inferior to the posterior axillary fold [21].

An incision along the anterior edge of the latissimus dorsi helps to identify the perforator [21]. In order to facilitate the intramuscular dissection, the posterior and inferior incisions are then finished. Perforator dissection continues until the horizontal and descending branches junction is met [21]. The pivot point, represented by this junction, is adequate enough to ensure proper closure of the axillary defect [21]. A flap as large as 15 × 8 cm can be based on this perforator (**Table 2**).

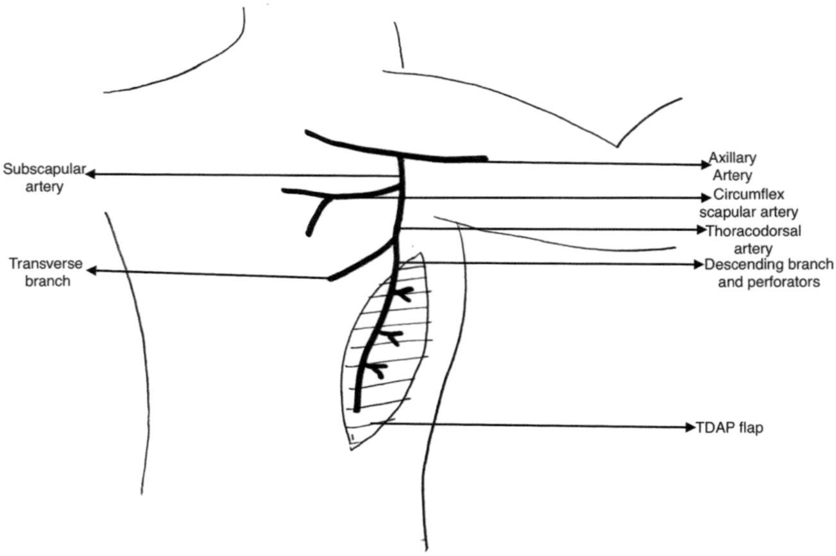

Figure 5.
Planning of thoracodorsal artery perforator flap.

Advantage	Disadvantages
It shares characteristics with the axilla due to its close anatomical proximity, such as adequate thickness and contour.	It requires microvascular skills for perforator dissection, and thus has steeper learning curve.
Its long pedicle allows for wide mobilization and cover of significant defects [20].	Extensive intramuscular dissection of the perforator is required to achieve a wider rotation arc.
There is no functional deficiency to the shoulder [20].	

Table 2.
Advantages and disadvantages of Thoracodorsal artery perforator (TDAP) flap.

3.1.3 Lateral thoracic artery perforator flap

With an extensive arc of rotation, the lateral thoracic region offers a dependable flap alternative (**Figure 6**). The axillary artery is the source vessel of the lateral thoracic artery. It provides a minor source of blood flow to the lateral thoracic wall and breast. Its perforators connect to those of the posterior intercostal vessels and the thoracodorsal system. These perforators are typically found lateral to the pectoralis major muscle on the anteroinferior edge of axilla [22]. The extent of the flap that can be raised safely is quite large, approximately 15 × 12 cm.

Between the pectoralis minor and latissimus dorsi muscles runs the lateral thoracic artery. Consequently, the flap is confined between the anterior and posterior axillary lines [22]. Depending on the required pedicle length, the pedicle can be dissected all the way up to the axillary artery [22]. Defects in the pectoral area, axilla, and proximal arm can be covered by the flap [22]. There are numerous angles at which the flap can be rotated, up to 180 degrees (**Table 3**).

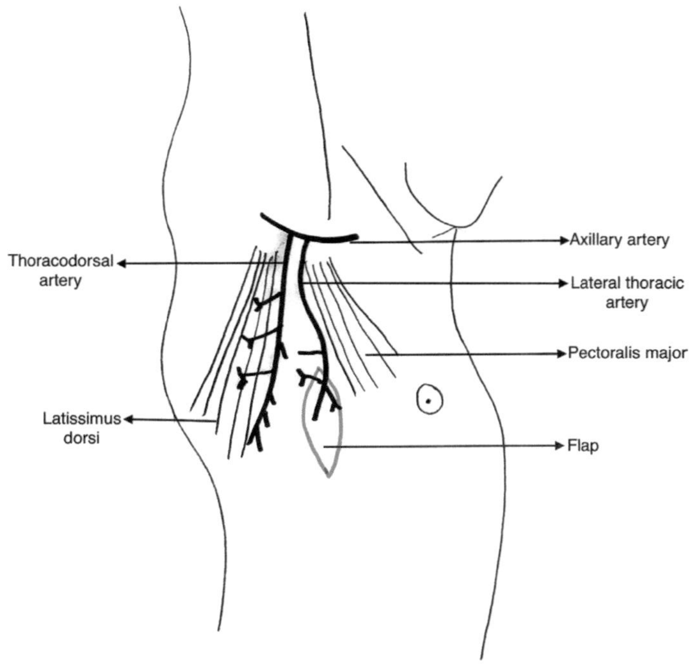

Figure 6.
Planning of lateral thoracic artery perforator flap.

Advantage	Disadvantages
The scar in the donor site is concealed.	The dissection is tedious.
There is no restriction of mobility of shoulder joint.	The location of perforators is variable.
	Donor site scar is, sometimes, visible on the anterolateral chest.

Table 3.
Advantages and disadvantages of Lateral thoracic artery perforator flap.

3.1.4 Posterior arm flap

An unnamed constant artery that emerges from the profunda brachii or brachial artery acts as vascular source of the flap. At the point of termination of the teres major tendon, the vessels pass through the triceps muscle aponeurosis [10].

The line that connects the posterior axillary fold with the olecranon acts as axis of the flap. A perforator is found 3–4 cm distal to the axillary crease of arm and 1–2 cm medial to the posterior axillary line. Up to the point where the proximal two thirds and distal one third of the arm meet, the largest flap can be raised. The flap width is the same as the amount of skin that can be closed primarily [10]. The flap is elevated up to the designated perforator in the subfascial plane.

The flap is elevated between the fascia and the triceps brachii muscle. On the deep surface of the flap, the pedicle is visible beneath the fascia. Either a peninsular flap or an islanded flap can be elevated. For the flap to reach the axillary defect, perforator dissection is not necessary [10, 23].

Advantage	Disadvantages
The flap skin is thin, pliable, and relatively hairless.	The blood supply is quite variable. In some cases, the artery may not be present and the flap would, then, be based on dermal blood supply and, thus, less reliable [19].
Donor scar is mostly concealed, in the inner aspect of the arm [19].	

Table 4.
Advantages and disadvantages of Posterior arm flap.

3.1.5 Medial arm flap

The superior ulnar collateral artery serves as the basis for the medial arm flap, which is an axial pattern flap. Originating 4–6 cm beyond the pectoralis major, the superior ulnar collateral artery is an axial cutaneous artery that travels distally through the subcutaneous tissue till it enters the medial arm skin 6–12 cm beyond the pectoralis [19]. Either the profunda brachii artery or the brachial artery directly branches out to form the superior ulnar collateral artery.

The proximally based medial arm flap extends from the mid-anterior to mid-posterior line [19]. Except in cases where the flap is extremely narrow, skin grafts are necessary to cover the donor site. Three-quarters of the length of the arm is the maximum length of the flap that may be raised safely. This length can be extended to the elbow by doing a delay procedure initially (**Table 4**) [19].

3.2 Inguinal and anogenital region

Defects in the groin and inguinal region are associated with greater morbidity and necessitate coverage with a flap, due to the following reasons:

- The inguinal region houses vital structures, such as femoral vessels, femoral nerve, and the great saphenous vein.
- There is potential for dead space in the region of the femoral triangle, with the presence of lymph nodes. Persistent raw areas in the inguinal region are complicated by lymphorrhoea, infection, and lymphangitis.
- This area is subjected to repeated tension during movement such as walking, sitting, squatting, and climbing stairs.
- This area is subjected to friction, both between the genitalia and thigh, and between the skin and clothes.

3.2.1 Tensor fascia lata (TFL) flap

For the restoration of defects in the inguinal and lower abdominal regions, the TFL fasciomyocutaneous flap is a versatile and robust choice [24]. Its vascular pedicle, the transverse branch of the lateral femoral circumflex artery has a constant anatomical course (**Figure 7**) [24]. The artery courses in between the vastus lateralis and the rectus femurs. Its transverse branch penetrates the TFL muscle. Between 8 and 12 cm

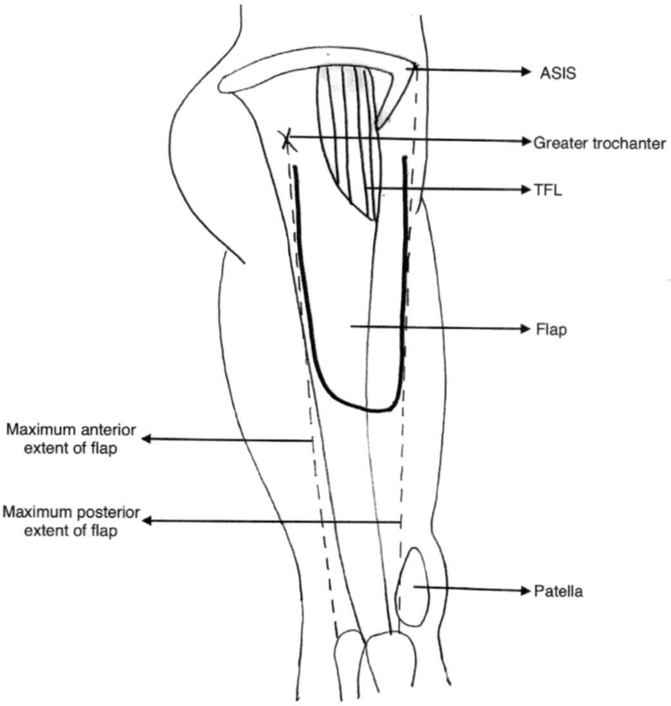

Figure 7.
Planning of TFL flap.

Advantage	Disadvantages
It has wide arc of rotation. Wider arc of rotation and the good length of the TFL flap can be utilized to cover defects in inguinal, anterior and posterior thigh, gluteal, and anogenital regions [25].	The flap is thin distally and bulky proximally. This creates an unsightly dog ear [25].
It has consistent vascular pedicle, good mobility and ease of positioning [25].	A significant amount of the thigh fat is taken with the flap, leading to contour differences and a depressed scar. This is more apparent when the donor area is grafted [25].
The donor site morbidity is low.	There may be a risk of weakness of knee and hip stability, which becomes significant in individuals, who have pre-existing hip and knee pathology.

Table 5.
Advantages and disadvantages of Tensor fascia lata (TFL) flap.

from the ASIS, the septocutaneous perforators emerge [25]. It is safe to raise a skin island up to 15 cm wide and around 8 cm above the knee [25]. If the flap breadth is less than 9 cm, the donor site can typically be closed primarily; otherwise, a skin graft may be used (**Table 5**) [25].

3.2.2 Anterolateral thigh (ALT) flap

For the lower abdomen and inguinal area, the ALT flap is a great choice [24]. Depending on the requirement, the flap can be raised using a variety of components,

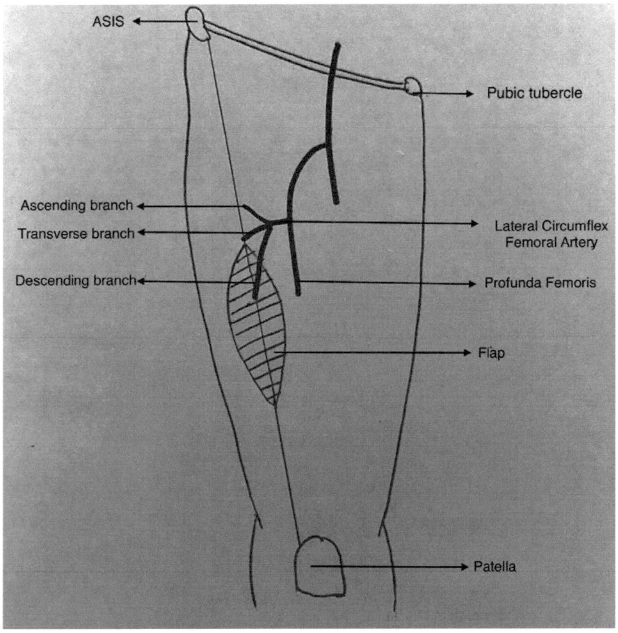

Figure 8.
Planning of anterolateral thigh flap.

including skin, subcutaneous fat, muscle, nerve, and fascia lata. It is based on perforators of the descending branch of lateral circumflex femoral artery (**Figure 8**) [24]. The surface marking of the intermuscular septum between the rectus femoris and vastus lateralis is represented by a line drawn from the anterior superior iliac spine to the superolateral edge of the patella. The flap perforators are mostly found in the area around the center of this line, with a radius of three to five centimeters [24]. A defect template is taken and positioned so that its arc of rotation of the provisionally

Advantage	Disadvantages
It has a long and constant pedicle, of 14–16 cm in length [24].	The risk of injury to motor nerve to vastus lateralis is real, as the nerve runs with the pedicle of this flap [25].
The flap skin is thin and pliable enough to be folded, tubed, or packed into cavities.	Cautious tunneling of the flap is required [25].
The flap harvest is easy [25].	
The flap has a vast skin territory.	
Even with a skin graft, the donor site is less conspicuous [25].	
The flap can be safely modified to a TFL or anteromedial thigh flap if the pedicle turns out to be missing [25].	
Coapting a nerve at the recipient site with the lateral or anterior cutaneous nerve of the thigh, which when raised with the flap can make the flap sensate [25].	

Table 6.
Advantages and disadvantages of Anterolateral thigh (ALT) flap.

chosen perforator reaches the defect. After raising the flap in a suprafascial or subfascial plane, pedicle is dissected proximally up to its origin [25]. Because of its close relationship to the vascular pedicle, the nerve to the vastus lateralis needs to be safeguarded [25].

Either above or deep to the rectus femoris and sartorius muscles, the flap is tunneled into the subcutaneous plane [24]. The donor site can be closed primarily or grafted depending on flap width. The flap can extend up to 8 cm over the perianal region, the whole groin, the contralateral lower abdomen, the contralateral inguinal area, and the umbilicus (**Table 6**).

3.2.3 Rectus abdominis myocutaneous flap - vertical (VRAM) or transverse (TRAM)

Defects in the axilla, lower chest, pelvis, perineum, groin, and proximal thigh can all be well treated with the pedicled rectus abdominis myocutaneous flap [25].

The muscle known as the rectus abdominis is vertically orientated and runs from the pubic ramus to the costal margins (**Figure 9**). Its blood supply comes from the Deep Superior epigastric artery and venae comitantes, as well as the Deep Inferior epigastric artery (DIEA) and venae comitantes. With an average size of 2.5–3.8 mm, the DIEA is the most prominent system [18]. However, the flap can typically survive on any of the two pedicles [25].

From the external iliac artery, just above the inguinal ligament, is the point where the DIEA begins. It then climbs obliquely to the posterior surface of the

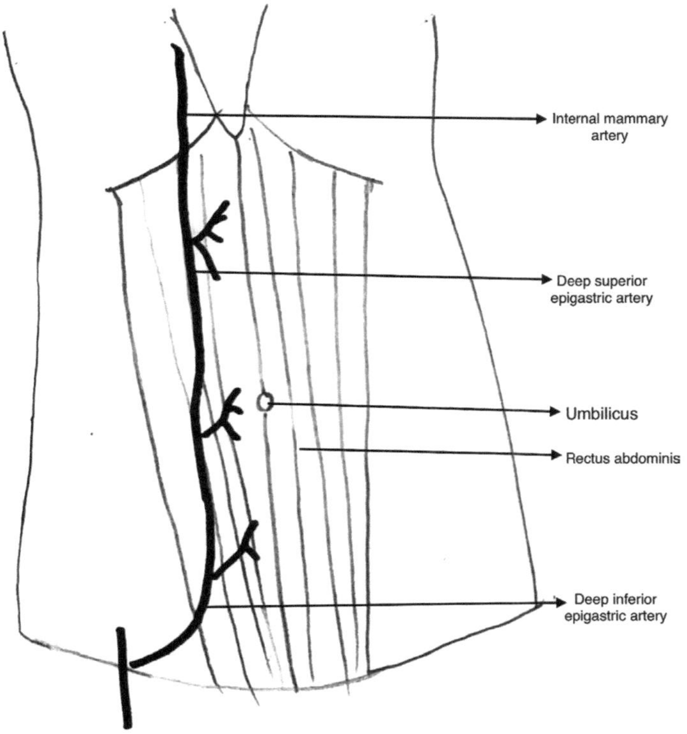

Figure 9.
Planning of vertical rectus abdominis flap.

Advantage	Disadvantages
It is a sturdy and versatile flap with a good arc of rotation which can reach diverse anatomical sites.	The harvest of anterior rectus sheath necessitates the application of mesh to prevent development of a hernia.
The flap harvest is easy.	
Raising of the flap does not warrant change in position of the patient.	
The flap can cover significant defects.	

Table 7.
Advantages and disadvantages of Rectus abdominis myocutaneous flap.

rectus abdominis muscle, about 7 cm above its insertion point [25]. The anterior rectus sheath is detected by laterally incising the skin paddle above the external oblique fascia [25]. The major trunk of the inferior epigastric vessels is skeletonized, and the vessels themselves can be seen and identified. The rectus muscle is incised superiorly and flap is raised off the posterior rectus sheath to inferior epigastric vessels. If necessary, an inferior cut over the rectus muscle may be made. The flap is then inserted into the defect after tunneling subcutaneously. To avoid a hernia, the anterior rectus fascia is closed. Mesh is used in closing if the tension is excessive (**Table 7**) [25].

3.2.4 Gracilis flap

The gracilis muscle flap can be utilized as a muscle flap with skin graft or as a myocutaneous flap [24]. The gracilis muscle is the most superficial adductor muscle of thigh region. It inserts on the medial surface of the tibia while originating from the inferior pubic ramus [19]. A branch of the medial circumflex femoral artery serves as the major source vessel [19]. It enters the deep aspect of the gracilis 8–10 cm distal to the pubic tubercle after passing between the adductor longus and adductor brevis muscles [19].

Additionally, the medial thigh skin, which covers the proximal two-thirds of the muscle and various quantities of surrounding skin, is supplied by the gracilis pedicle [19]. The semitendinosus tendon at the knee and the pubic tubercle are connected in a straight line. It is best to design the skin paddle posterior to the line. The skin island may typically be reliably raised to a maximum size of 22 × 8 cm (**Table 8**).

Advantage	Disadvantages
Harvest of the flap leaves no noticeable functional loss.	There is limited arc of rotation due to limited pedicle length.
Donor site is amenable to primary closure.	
Relatively concealed donor scars on the inner thigh	
The vascular pedicle is of large caliber and long enough, consistently located, and easily dissected.	

Table 8.
Advantages and disadvantages of Gracilis flap.

3.2.5 Rectus femoris flap

Reconstruction of the lower abdominal wall, perineum, and trochanteric areas is possible with the rectus femoris flap because of its extensive arc of rotation [19]. The most anterior muscle in the quadriceps group, the rectus femoris, originates from the anterior superior iliac spine and inserts into the patellar tendon in tandem with the vastus lateralis, medialis, and intermedius [25]. About 6 cm above the patella, the muscle fibers end and forms the tendon (**Figure 10**).

The descending branch of lateral femoral circumflex artery serves as the vascular supply. In the proximal part of the muscle, three to four perforators originate. The skin of anterior third thigh is supplied by the same perforators. Safe harvesting of flaps up to 15 × 40 cm has been accomplished. If the skin island is less than 6 cm in width, the donor site is amenable to primary closure [19]. The muscle rotates around the neurovascular pedicle, which is roughly 8 cm away from the inguinal ligament [19].

Loss of strength in the knee extension is the limiting factor preventing widespread use of this flap [24]. There can be a 24–28% reduction in quadriceps strength after raising this muscle as a flap, limiting the usefulness of this flap (**Table 9**) [25].

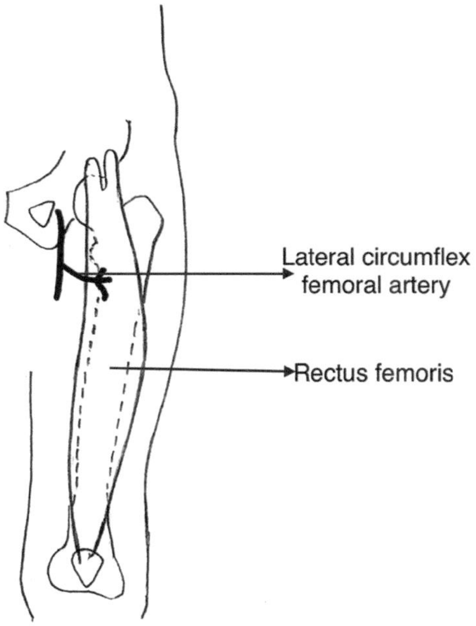

Figure 10.
Planning of rectus femoris flap.

Advantage	Disadvantages
A large skin island can be raised.	There is a reduction in the strength of knee extension.

Table 9.
Advantages and disadvantages of rectus femoris flap.

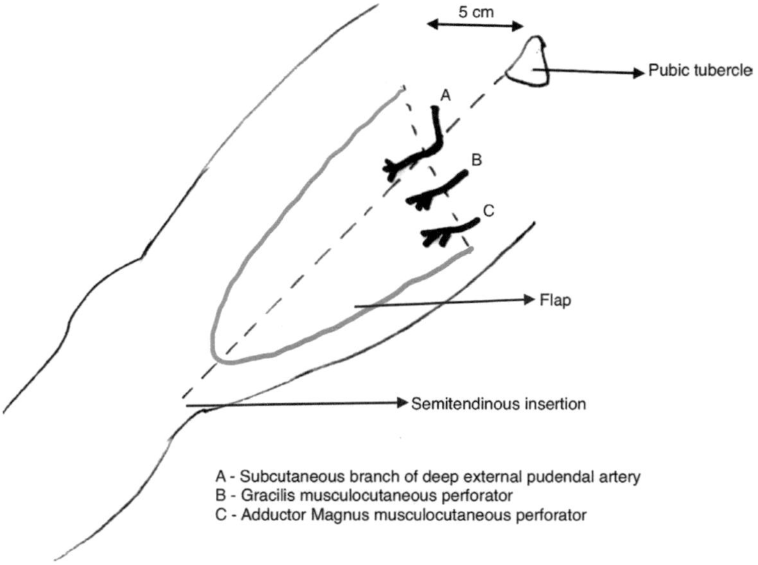

Figure 11.
Planning of medial thigh flap.

3.2.6 Medial thigh flap

The medial thigh flap is a long, narrow, fasciocutaneous flap with a wide arc of rotation [19]. It allows transfer of large skin islands for total scrotal, groin, or perineal defects [19].

Indirect branches from the musculocutaneous perforators of the adductor compartment and the external pudendal vessels or septocutaneous branches of the superficial femoral or medial circumflex femoral arteries provide circulation to the flap (**Figure 11**) [19]. When a line is traced from the pubic tubercle to the ischial ramus, these perforators are located within 5 cm [19].

The anterior edge of the flap is indicated by a line drawn from the pubic tubercle to the semitendinosus tendon insertion [19]. The posterior margin is determined by pinching the thigh. Wider the flap, more perforators are included, thus ensuring safety of a longer flap. Up to 20 cm long flap can be raised safely.

3.3 Propeller flaps

The propeller flap is raised as an islanded flap. The feeding vascular pedicle serves as the pivot point, and it is shaped like a propeller blade with two blades of uneven length (**Figure 12**). The short arm completely or partially covers the donor defect when the blades are propelled or switched, while the long arm covers the defect. The flap has a 180-degree rotational range. It is a very adaptable flap because it can draw tissues from nearby non-traumatized regions. Propeller flaps are not constrained by the length-to-width ratio guidelines [26]. For covering defects of the axilla, propeller flaps can be based on the above-mentioned perforators from either the medial arm or the lateral chest wall. For covering defects of inguinal area, perforators from medial thigh or groin may be used.

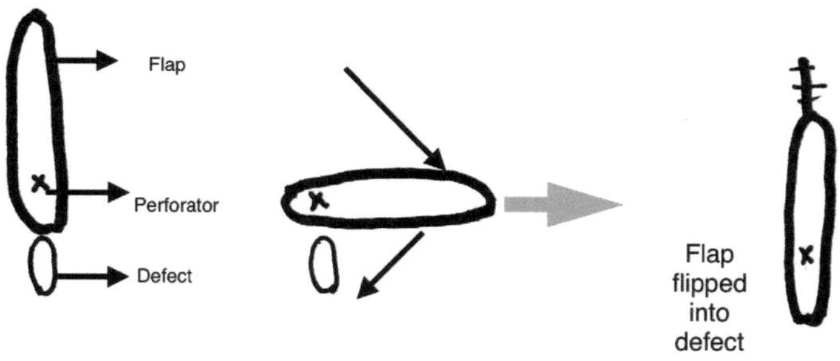

Figure 12.
Planning of propeller flap.

4. Dermal substitutes

In the early 1980s, Burke et al. initially reported using a collagen-glycosaminoglycan scaffold for treating cutaneous defects [27]. Initially, dermal templates were used in extensive burn injuries where donor skin was limited. In the present era, their clinical applications have broadened significantly. They provide a soft tissue platform and, once integrated, are amenable to grafting. Dermal substitutes are used to improve functional and esthetic outcomes [27].

Integra®, the first commercially available skin substitute, is a collagen type I cross-linked matrix made of glycosaminoglycans obtained from cows. It resembles the dermal structure of humans. A silicone film covers it, briefly simulating the function of the epidermis [27]. The vascularized wound bed is treated with Integra®. In 2 to 3 weeks, a vascularized neodermis is formed as blood vessels and cells proliferate into the collagen matrix [27]. After revascularization is complete, a small skin graft is placed after the silicone layer is removed. Following the development of Integra®, a number of other dermal replacements derived from humans and animals are currently marketed.

MatriDerm®, a collagen matrix developed from cows that has non-crosslinked collagen fibers of types I, III, and V and is coated with elastin fibers, is another artificially created dermal substitute [27]. Permanent dermal-regenerating templates, such as Integra® and MatriDerm®, are synthetic dermal substitutes that are eventually covered by an epidermal autologous graft [27]. Various other skin substitutes that are available, but not popular in our country, are Biobrane®, Alloderm®, Transcyte®, Dermagraft®, and Apligraf®.

5. Conclusion

Patients with hidradenitis suppurativa already experience a significant decline in their quality of life. Reconstruction of high quality is individualized, reproducible, and reliable. Basic flaps must be part of the armamentarium of all surgeons treating hidradenitis suppurativa. This chapter serves as a guide to understanding the requirements of the defect, as well as designing and executing an appropriate flap.

Acknowledgements

The authors acknowledge the Department of Plastic Surgery, AIIMS Jodhpur.

Conflict of interest

The authors declare no conflict of interest.

Author details

Shilpi Karmakar* and Ramani Saradha
Department of Burns and Plastic Surgery, All India Institute of Medical Sciences, Jodhpur, Rajasthan, India

*Address all correspondence to: drshilpikarmakar@rediffmail.com

References

[1] Vaillant C, Berkane Y, Lupon E, Atlan M, Rousseau P, Lellouch AG, et al. Outcomes and reliability of perforator flaps in the reconstruction of hidradenitis Suppurativa defects: A systemic review and meta-analysis. Journal of Clinical Medicine. 2022;**11**:5813. DOI: 10.3390/jcm11195813

[2] Miller A, Shahzeidi P, Bernhardt M. An update on current clinical management and emerging treatments in hidradenitis Suppurativa. Skin Therapy Letter. 2024;**29**:1-6

[3] Danby FW, Hazen PG, Boer J. New and traditional surgical approaches to hidradenitis suppurativa. Journal of the American Academy of Dermatology. 2015;**73**:S62-S65. DOI: 10.1016/j.jaad.2015.07.043

[4] Navrazhina K, Frew JW, Gilleaudeau P, Sullivan-Whalen M, Garcet S, Krueger JG. Epithelialized tunnels are a source of inflammation in hidradenitis suppurativa. The Journal of Allergy and Clinical Immunology. 2021;**147**:2213-2224. DOI: 10.1016/j.jaci.2020.12.651

[5] Kim ES, Garnock-Jones KP, Keam SJ. Adalimumab: A review in hidradenitis suppurativa. American Journal of Clinical Dermatology. 2016;**17**:545-552. DOI: 10.1007/s40257-016-0220-6

[6] Kimball AB, Okun MM, Williams DA, et al. Two phase 3 trials of adalimumab for hidradenitis suppurativa. The New England Journal of Medicine. 2016;**375**:422-434. DOI: 10.1056/NEJMoa1504370

[7] Jemec GBE, Okun MM, Forman SB, et al. Adalimumab medium-term dosing strategy in moderate-to-severe hidradenitis suppurativa: Integrated results from the phase III randomized placebo-controlled PIONEER trials. The British Journal of Dermatology. 2019;**181**:967-975. DOI: 10.1111/bjd.17919

[8] Nazzaro G, Calzari P, Vaienti S, Passoni E, Marzano AV. The role of imaging technologies in the diagnosis of hidradenitis suppurativa. Clinics in Dermatology. 2023;**41**:611-621. DOI: 10.1016/j.clindermatol.2023.08.023

[9] Marasca C, Marasca D, Megna M, Annunziata MC, Fabbrocini G. Ultrasound: An indispensable tool to evaluate the outcome of surgical approaches in patients affected by hidradenitis suppurativa. Journal of the European Academy of Dermatology and Venereology. 2020;**34**:e413-e414. DOI: 10.1111/jdv.16361

[10] Kingsly PM, Ete G, Felix Cordelia MJ, Akamanchi AK, Agarwal S. Simultaneous bilateral reconstruction of the axilla with posterior arm flap in recurrent hidradenitis suppurativa. The Indian Journal of Plastic Surgery. 2022;**55**(1):66-69. Published 2022 Feb 16. DOI: 10.1055/s-0041-1740087

[11] Marchesi A, Marcelli S, Zingaretti N, Parodi PC, Vaienti L. Pedicled thoracodorsal artery perforator and muscle-sparing latissimus Dorsi flaps in the axillary reconstruction after hidradenitis Suppurativa excision: Functional and aesthetic issues. Annals of Plastic Surgery. 2018;**81**:694-701. DOI: 10.1097/SAP.0000000000001664

[12] Revol M, Servant JM. Techniques Chirurgicales—Chirurgie Plastique Reconstructrice et Esthétique. Volume 5. Round Rock, TX, USA: EMC; 2010. Cicatrisation Dirigée

[13] Ovadja ZN, Zugaj M, Jacobs W, van der Horst CMAM, Lapid O. Recurrence rates following reconstruction strategies after wide excision of hidradenitis suppurativa: A systematic review and meta-analysis. Dermatologic Surgery. 2021;**47**:e106-e110. DOI: 10.1097/DSS.0000000000002815

[14] Deckers IE, Dahi Y, van der Zee HH, Prens EP. Hidradenitis suppurativa treated with wide excision and second intention healing: A meaningful local cure rate after 253 procedures. Journal of the European Academy of Dermatology and Venereology. 2018;**32**:459-462. DOI: 10.1111/jdv.14770

[15] Wormald JCR, Balzano A, Clibbon JJ, Figus A. Surgical treatment of severe hidradenitis suppurativa of the axilla: Thoracodorsal artery perforator (TDAP) flap versus split skin graft. Journal of Plastic, Reconstructive & Aesthetic Surgery. 2014;**67**:1118-1124. DOI: 10.1016/j.bjps.2014.04.032

[16] Starkman SJ, Williams CT, Sherris DA. Flap basics I: Rotation and transposition flaps. Facial Plastic Surgery Clinics of North America. 2017;**25**:313-321. DOI: 10.1016/j.fsc.2017.03.004

[17] Sharma RK, Krishnan MK, Singh G. Reconstruction in extensive axillary hidradenitis suppurativa with local fasciocutaneous V-Y advancement flaps. The Indian Journal of Plastic Surgery. 2006;**39**:18-21. DOI: 10.1055/s-0039-1700454

[18] Mandal A, Watson J. Experience with different treatment modules in hidradenitis suppuritiva: A study of 106 cases. The Surgeon. 2005;**3**:23-26. DOI: 10.1016/s1479-666x(05)80006-x

[19] Khayat S, Bonsfills N, Antunez-Conde R, Alvarez-Mokthari S, Aranibar H, Tousidonis M, et al. Parascapular flap for severe hidradenitis suppurativa. Case Reports in Dermatology. 2024;**16**:8-16. DOI: 10.1159/000533387

[20] Busnardo FF, Coltro PS, Olivan MV, Busnardo APV, Ferreira MC. The thoracodorsal artery perforator flap in the treatment of axillary hidradenitis suppurativa: Effect on preservation of arm abduction. Plastic and Reconstructive Surgery. 2011;**128**:949-953. DOI: 10.1097/PRS.0b013e3182268c38

[21] Ortiz CL, Castillo VL, Pilarte FS, Barraguer EL. Experience using the thoracodorsal artery perforator flap in axillary hidradentitis suppurativa cases. Aesthetic Plastic Surgery. 2010;**34**:785-792. DOI: 10.1007/s00266-010-9544-4

[22] Baghaki S, Cevirme M, Diyarbakirli M, Tatar C, Aydin Y. Locoregional use of lateral thoracic artery perforator flap as a propeller flap. Annals of Plastic Surgery. 2015;**74**:532-535. DOI: 10.1097/SAP.0000000000000516

[23] Hodgins N, Bhat W, Pape SA. The posterior arm flap in reconstruction of axillary defects: A lifeboat when soft tissue cover is limited. Journal of Plastic, Reconstructive & Aesthetic Surgery. 2015;**68**:1629-1631. DOI: 10.1016/j.bjps.2015.07.011

[24] Azevedo RA, Roxo AC, Alvares SHB, Baptista DP, Favorito LA. Use of flaps in inguinal lymphadenectomy in metastatic penile cancer. International Brazilian Journal of Urology. 2021;**47**:1108-1119. DOI: 10.1590/S1677-5538.IBJU.2021.99.14

[25] Murthy V, Gopinath KS. Reconstruction of groin defects following radical inguinal lymphadenectomy: An evidence based review. Indian Journal of Surgical Oncology. 2012;**3**:130-138. DOI: 10.1007/s13193-012-0145-3

[26] Ono S, Sebastin SJ, Yazaki N, Hyakusoku H, Chung KC. Clinical 22 applications of perforator-based propeller flaps in upper limb soft tissue reconstruction. The Journal of Hand Surgery. 2011;**36**:853-863. DOI: 10.1016/j.jhsa.2010.12.021

[27] Rehim SA, Singhal M, Chung KC. Dermal skin substitutes for upper limb reconstruction: Current status, indications, and contraindications. Hand Clinics. 2014;**30**(239-52):vii. DOI: 10.1016/j.hcl.2014.02.001